Al-Mamun
Taksim Ahmed
Sukalyan Kumar Kundu

# Metronidazole Extended Release Solid Dosage Form

Md. Abdullah- Al-Mamun
Taksim Ahmed
Sukalyan Kumar Kundu

# Metronidazole Extended Release Solid Dosage Form

Development of extended release formulation and in vitro bioequivalence study of Metronidazole solid dosage form

LAP LAMBERT Academic Publishing

**Impressum / Imprint**

Bibliografische Information der Deutschen Nationalbibliothek: Die Deutsche Nationalbibliothek verzeichnet diese Publikation in der Deutschen Nationalbibliografie; detaillierte bibliografische Daten sind im Internet über http://dnb.d-nb.de abrufbar.

Alle in diesem Buch genannten Marken und Produktnamen unterliegen warenzeichen-, marken- oder patentrechtlichem Schutz bzw. sind Warenzeichen oder eingetragene Warenzeichen der jeweiligen Inhaber. Die Wiedergabe von Marken, Produktnamen, Gebrauchsnamen, Handelsnamen, Warenbezeichnungen u.s.w. in diesem Werk berechtigt auch ohne besondere Kennzeichnung nicht zu der Annahme, dass solche Namen im Sinne der Warenzeichen- und Markenschutzgesetzgebung als frei zu betrachten wären und daher von jedermann benutzt werden dürften.

Bibliographic information published by the Deutsche Nationalbibliothek: The Deutsche Nationalbibliothek lists this publication in the Deutsche Nationalbibliografie; detailed bibliographic data are available in the Internet at http://dnb.d-nb.de.

Any brand names and product names mentioned in this book are subject to trademark, brand or patent protection and are trademarks or registered trademarks of their respective holders. The use of brand names, product names, common names, trade names, product descriptions etc. even without a particular marking in this works is in no way to be construed to mean that such names may be regarded as unrestricted in respect of trademark and brand protection legislation and could thus be used by anyone.

Coverbild / Cover image: www.ingimage.com

Verlag / Publisher:
LAP LAMBERT Academic Publishing
ist ein Imprint der / is a trademark of
AV Akademikerverlag GmbH & Co. KG
Heinrich-Böcking-Str. 6-8, 66121 Saarbrücken, Deutschland / Germany
Email: info@lap-publishing.com

Herstellung: siehe letzte Seite /
Printed at: see last page
ISBN: 978-3-659-35589-9

Zugl. / Approved by: Bangladesh, Jahangirnagar University, Diss., 2009

# CONTENTS

## LIST OF TABLES

## LIST OF FIGURES

# Abstract

## Development of extended release formulation and in vitro bioequivalence study of Metronidazole solid dosage form.

In the present study, an attempt was made to develop an extended release metronidazole composition that will be capable of delivering acceptable bioavailability for up to 24 hours. For this purpose Eudragit NM30D and Methocel Premium K4M were used as retardant material. Using various proportions of Eudragit NM30D and Methocel Premium K4M, extended release formulations of Metronidazole were prepared separately through wet granulation. Three formulations (U-1 to U-3) were developed using Eudragit NM30D as release retardant and while another five (M-1 to M-5) using Methocel Premium K4M. The granules for tabletting were evaluated for moisture content, loose bulk density, tapped bulk density, compressibility index, angle of repose etc. Tablets were subjected to thickness, hardness and friability and in vitro release studies. Dissolution study of formulations of Eudragit NM30D and Methocel K4M based tablet matrices were carried out in 0.1 N Hydrochloric acid for 12 hours period. The granules showed satisfactory flow properties, compressibility index and drug content etc. All the tablets complied with pharmacopoeial specifications. The dissolution data were treated by Zero-order, First-order, Higuchi, and Korsmeyer-Peppas equation. The regression coefficients were used to determine the release kinetics for both polymer matrices. Dissolution profiles of proposed formulations were compared with Innovator drug in term of Difference Factor ($f_1$) and Similarity factor ($f_2$). It was observed that formulation U-1, U-2, M-2, M-3, M-4 meet the specification of bioequibalance with Flagyl ER in terms of Difference

11

Factor ($f_1$) and Similarity Factor ($f_2$) among them M-3 showed the highest similarity and lowest difference factor with the innovators' drug Flagyl ER. Three bathes of the formulation M-3 were prepared which were then studied for accelerated stability testing of six months.

## 1. Introduction

Research and development of drug delivery systems are increasing at a rapid pace throughout the world. This worldwide trend will intensify in the next decade as cuts in public health expenses demand lower costs and higher efficacy. The fundamental target of any drug delivery system is to provide a therapeutic amount of drug to the proper site in the body to achieve promptly and then maintain the desired drug concentration for a definite period of time. Depending on the route of administration, a conventional dosage form of the drug e.g. solution, suspension, capsule, tablet etc produce a drug blood level time profile which does not maintain within the therapeutic range for extended period of time. The short duration of action is due to the inability of the conventional dosage forms to control temporal delivery. If any attempt is made to maintain drug blood level in the therapeutic range for longer periods by, for example increasing the dose of an intravenous injection, toxic levels may be produced at any time. An alternative is to administer the drug repetitively using a constant dosing interval as in multiple dosing therapies. In this case drug blood level reached and the time required reaching that level depends on the dose and the dosing interval. There are some potential problems inherent to multiple dose therapy. First if the dosing interval is not appropriate for the biological half life of the drug, large peaks and valleys in the drug blood level may result. Secondly the drug blood level may not be with in the

12

therapeutic range at sufficiently early times, an important consideration for certain disease states. Thirdly patient noncompliance with the multiple dosing regimens can result in the failure of the approach. In recent years considerable attention has been focused on the development of new drug delivery systems. Recognition of the possibility of re-patenting successful drugs by applying the concepts and techniques of controlled release drug delivery systems, coupled with the increasing expense in bringing new drug entities to market, has encouraged the development of new drug delivery systems. Therapeutic efficacy & safety of drugs administered by conventional methods can be improved by more precise spatial and temporal placement within the body, thereby reducing both the size and number of doses.

Ideally, a thorough understanding of each of these stages for a given drug is essential for achieving its most effective therapeutic efficacy in patients. The pharmaceutical phase describes the process of a drug's conversion from a chemical form into a dosage form. This phase includes the characterization of physicochemical drug profiles, design and production of dosage forms, and biopharmaceutical evaluation of drug products. The pharmaceutical phase can initially influence the pharmacokinetic phase, which is measured by blood-level-versus-time profiles. The pharmacokinetic phase then directly affects the pharmacodynamic or efficacy phase. Modern drugs are rarely administered in pure chemical form. Rather, they are prepared in a vehicle called a drug delivery system. The goal of any drug delivery system is to provide a therapeutic amount of drug to the proper site in the body to achieve the desired drug concentration. That is, the drug-delivery system should deliver drug at a rate dictated by the needs of the body over the period of treatment. This idealized objective points to the two aspects most important to drug delivery, namely, spatial placement and temporal delivery of a drug. Spatial placement relates to targeting a drug to a specific organ or tissue, while temporal delivery refers to controlling the rate of drug delivery to the target tissue. The bulk of research has been directed at oral dosage forms that satisfy the temporal aspect of drug delivery, but many of the newer approaches under investigation may allow for spatial placement as well.

## 1.1 Categories of Drug Delivery System

Depending on the route of administration and therapeutic objectives, the drug delivery systems can be categorized as-

**a) Conventional drug delivery systems:**

     i. Solids

     ii. Liquids

     iii. Semisolids

**b) Controlled-release drug delivery systems:**

     i. Sustained release

     ii. Prolonged release

     iii. Pulse-release

     iv. Constant release

**c) Novel drug delivery systems:**

     I. Targeted

     II. Self-regulated

     III. Biofeedback

     IV. Biological carriers

Most conventional dosage forms function merely to place a drug at the site of administration and pay no regard to the regulation of release and absorption or the duration and targeting of drug in the body. So now a day's one of the most active areas of research and development in drug delivery involves "controlled release" products rather than develop new drug entities at great cost; as some drug therapies already on the market can be improved simply by controlling the rate at which they enter the blood stream.

Joseph R. Robinson has claimed in the book **'Sustained and controlled release drug delivery systems'** that-

"............drug delivery must be continued at a rate such that the condition in question is cured or controlled in a minimum time with the fewest side effects. Thus, an appropriate definition of controlled drug release is as follows: It is the phasing of drug administration to the needs of the condition at hand so that an optimal amount of drug is used to cure or control the condition in a minimum time. In some situations this might mean that drug is delivered more promptly for short periods of time and in other cases it would mean prolongation of drug levels. In the latter category we employ the terms 'sustained release' and 'prolonged release' interchangeably; this designates only one aspect of controlled release , namely, to produce protracted levels of drug in the body.............."

## 1.2 Extended Release Dosage Form (SRDF) Concept

Before initiating a discussion of extended and controlled release dosage forms, it is necessary to provide a short explanation of terminology. The general consensus is that control release denotes systems which can provide some control, whether this is of a temporal or spatial nature, or both, of drug in body. In other words, the system attempts to control drug concentration in the target tissue or cells. Thus prolong release or sustain release systems which only prolong therapeutic blood or tissue levels of the drug for an extended period of time, can't be considered as control

15

release systems by this definition. They are distinguished rate controlled drug delivery systems which are able to specify the release rate and duration in vivo precisely. Drug targeting on the other hand can be considered as a form of controlled release in that it exercises spatial control of drug release within the body.

In general controlled delivery attempts to:

a) Sustain drug action at a predetermined rate by maintaining a relatively constant, effective drug level in the body with concomitant minimization of undesirable side effects associated with a saw tooth kinetic pattern.

b) Localize drug action by spatial placement of a controlled release system (usually rate-controlled) adjacent to or in the diseased tissue or organ.

c) Target drug action by using carriers or chemical derivation to deliver drug to a particular "target" cell type.

Sustain release dosage forms include those dosage forms in which the drug-release characteristics are different from the conventional dosage form to saw-tooth pattern of drug delivery (Except continuous IV perfusion) & results in increase adverse effects, decrease therapeutic effect & poor patient compliance (Madan, 1990).

The USP defines modified release dosage form as "One for which the drug-release characteristics of time-course and/ or location are chosen to accomplish therapeutic of convenience objectives not offered by conventional dosage forms". At present time USP recognizes and defines only two types of modified release dosage forms: "Extended release" and Delayed release".

An 'extended-release' dosage is defined as "One that allows at least a two-fold reduction in dosing frequency as compared to that drug presented as a conventional solid dosage form". A delayed-release dosage form is defined as 'One that a drug(s) at a time other than promptly after administration'.

Sustain- release systems include any drug delivery system that achieves slow release of drug over an extended period of time. If the system is successful at maintaining constant drug levels in the blood or target tissue, it is considered a controlled-release system. If it is unsuccessful at this, but nevertheless the duration of action over that achieved by conventional delivery, it is considered a prolonged-release system.

According to Ballard, (1978), Extended release, extended action, prolonged action, controlled release, extended action, time release, depot, and repository dosage forms are termed used to identify drug delivery systems that are designed to achieve a prolonged therapeutic effect by continuously releasing medication over an extended period of time after administration of single dose. In the case of such dosage forms, this period may vary from days to months. In the case of orally administered forms, however, this period is measured in hours and critically depends on the residence time of the dosage form in the gastro intestinal tract.The rate of absorption of a drug from a dosage form can be decreased by reducing the rate of release of drug from the dosage form. When a drug is administered, after a certain time a peak blood level is attained which immediately begins to fall as the drug is eliminated or detoxified.

The products that are designed for the purpose of prolonged action by controlling the rate of release of drug over an extended period of time and ultimately maintaining this response at the initial level for ten to twelve hours or in some case for several days, weeks or even months, are termed as extended action (release) dosage form.

## 1.3 Synonyms of Extended Release Dosage Form

Many terms are used to describe modified-release products including

- Sustained release dosage form
- Prolonged release dosage form
- Delayed release dosage form
- Controlled release dosage form
- Timed release dosage form
- Retarded dosage form
- Extended action dosage form
- Depot dosage form
- Repeat dosage form
- Repository dosage form

In general, these terms are interchangeable.

There are three main categories of controlled drug release systems (Juliano, 1980):

**a) Extended drug action**

The systemic drug level far exceeds the therapeutic level for a brief period after ingestion or injection (in typical cases). The drug level then gradually declines from therapeutic to ineffective levels. This is an undesirable effect, especially when the therapeutic and toxic levels of a drug are close (that is the therapeutic index is low). Controlled drug delivery can help reduce this "sawtooth" profile. The flip side of reducing negative effects is the promotion of positive effects. Controlled drug delivery can also be used to provide a consistent and extended dosage. The therapeutic effectiveness of certain drugs can be greatly improved through sustaining an appropriate level of the drugs over time.

**b) Localized drug action**

It is often desirable to confine the action of a drug to a particular diseased tissue or organ without system wide (adverse) effects. For example, anticancer, antifertility and anti-inflammatory applications. Again, taking the positive viewpoint, localization can also enhance the therapeutic effectiveness of a drug. For example, intraocular treatment for glaucoma.

## c) Targeting drug action

The ideal form of DDS would be the "magic bullet" envisioned by the 1908 Nobel Laureate Paul Ehrlich. According to the Nobel Museum:

"His aim was, as he put it, to find chemical substances which have special affinities for pathogenic organisms, to which they would go, as antitoxins go to the toxins to which they are specifically related, and would be, as Ehrlich expressed it, `magic bullets' which would go straight to the organisms at which they were aimed". This would require the development of pharmaceutical products that would at least equal the effectiveness of natural "effectors". It should be noted that there is a distinction between targeting and localization. Localization means confining the drug to an organ or space in the body, while targeting involves more subtle action where the drug affects particular cell types.

Complicating the need for self-administered, targeted, extended release with increased bioavailability is the need to improve patient compliance. To achieve improved compliance will require further simplification of the user experience. The next step can easily be envisioned as involving further integration of devices and drugs to provide means to deliver multiple therapies in a simple, pain free, unobtrusive and targeted extended release device. The proper combination of technology portfolios, intellectual property, market and stakeholder understanding required achieve this next step is the challenge on the horizon. The goal/objective of any drug delivery system is to provide a therapeutic amount of drug to the proper site in the body to achieve promptly, and then maintain, the desired drug concentration. This idealized objective points to the two aspects most important to drug delivery, namely, spatial placement and temporal delivery of a drug. Spatial placement relates to targeting a drug to a specific organ or tissue while temporal delivery refers to controlling the rate of drug delivery to the target tissue. An appropriately designed extended-release drug delivery system can be a major advance toward solving these two problems (Longer *et al.*, 1990*)*. So the Drug Delivery Scientists have directed their research activities towards an oral dosage forms that satisfy the temporal aspect of drug delivery and new strategic innovation are under investigation that may allow for spatial placement as well.

The expanding arena of emerging drugs combined with increased sensitivity to clinical outcomes and healthcare costs and driving the need for alternative drug delivery methods and devices. More and more, the development of drugs and the development of delivery systems are being integrated to optimize the efficacy and cost- effectiveness of the therapy. In this concept, the extended or controlled release dosage forms have been designed with a view to deliver the drug at a rate directed by the needs of the body over the period of treatment. This may necessitate the delivery to occur at a constant rate for drugs that have a clear relationship between steady state plasma levels and the resultant therapeutic response or at a variable rate for drugs that need either a series of peaks and valleys or act in rhythm. Technologies are being developed to control drug release that will ensure efficient drug absorption and enhanced bioavailability.

## 1.4    History and Modern Development of Modified Release Dosage Forms

The modern era can be marked from WWII (1934 - 1944) approximately. Pharmaceutical firms developed with a primary mission of consistency in the preparation of dosage forms (drug delivery systems). The first extended release dosage form was marketed in the United States in 1952 by Smith Kline & French under the trade name 'Dexadrin Spansule'. The Spansule provided a novel form of drug delivery and was a major therapeutic breakthrough. It quickly released the required initial dose and then slowly and gradually released many extremely small doses to maintain a therapeutic level lasting from 10 to 12 hours, providing all-day or all-night therapy with one dose. The goal behind the development of oral controlled-release formulations at that time was the achievement of a constant release rate of the entrapped drug. On the basis of that concept, the zero-order osmotic delivery used in Procardia XL became one of the top 10 best selling medicines in the past century.

In 1968, Alejandro Zaffaroni founded ALZA (ALZA, 2003), now owned by Johnson and Johnson with the aim of creating controlled drug delivery systems whose release rate of drug could be controlled with precision, independent of the release environment. The formation of ALZA marked the beginning of the modern era of drug delivery technology (Robinson, 1978). And Elan Corporation was founded in 1969 "with a vision: to approach the challenge of drug delivery from an entirely new angle - that of controlled absorption of a drug to provide longer duration of drug effect".

Two major disease groups that have had an important bearing on the evolving nature of controlled drug delivery:

1. Diabetes - fluctuations in insulin/glucose minimized [extended drug release]

21

2. Cancer - target abnormal cells [localized / targeted drug release]

From an economic point of view, the development of novel delivery systems can potentially prove profitable for a modest investment (in terms of acquiring market share). In Time magazine of Jan. 13th this year, Charles P. Wallace wrote: "R and D costs as a percentage of drug-company sales were 12% in 1970, 15% in 1990 and 20% today". According to Visiongain, revenues of pharma products that utilize advanced drug delivery technology were estimated at US$38 billion in 2002. The growth of this market is expected to continue at an average rate of 28% over the next 5 years, significantly higher than the pace of the overall industry (Corporate Fact Sheet, Q2 2005, www.mistralpharma.com).Recently Controlled drug delivery industries have made certain gold standard innovation in drug delivery technology. Ms. Callanan commented, "Definitely a key for large pharma companies is to use novel approaches to extend the patent life of their products or, even if they don't extend the patent life, to add something new to the compound to get marketing advantage. Things like fast-melt technology, extended release compounds, all those areas, those types of technologies; in the next few years they will be exploited to their fullest extent by large pharma companies to protect their compounds  on the market." The majority of oral drug delivery systems are matrix-based.  Erosion, diffusion and swelling of the matrix are the various methods through which the systems control drug delivery. The swellable matrices are monolithic systems prepared by compressing a powdered mixture of a hydrophilic polymer and a drug (Hogan, 1989). The hydrophilic matrices are and interesting option when developing an oral extended-release formulation. The release of drug from such matrices can be controlled through their physical properties, the correct choice of gelling agent and setting up the conditions for fabrication (Vezquez *et al.*, 1995). The future of controlled release products is promising especially in the areas of Chronopharmacokinetic systems and Mucoadhesive delivery (Amidon and Löbenberg, 2000).

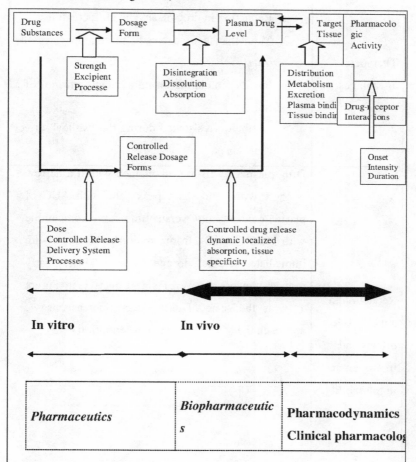

Figure 1.1: Flow diagram showing the path followed by a drug administered in either conventional or controlled-release formulations to its site of therapeutic action (Chien YW, 1992).

## 1.5 Advantages of Modified Release Dosage Forms

**Table 1.1: Benefit characteristics of modified release dosage forms**

| Benefit | Reasons |
|---|---|
| Therapeutic advantages | 1. Reduce the total amount of drug required.<br>2. Reduction in drug plasma level fluctuations;<br>3. Maintenance of a steady plasma level of the drug<br>4. Ideally simulating an intravenous infusion of a drug.<br>5. Antibiotic resistance during the "valley" effect is absent |
| Reduction in adverse side effects and improvement in tolerability | Drug plasma levels are maintained within a narrow window with no sharp peaks and with AUC of plasma concentration versus time curve comparable with total AUC from multiple dosing with immediate release dosage forms. This greatly reduces the possibility of side effects (see Figure 1.2), as the scale of side effects increase as we approach the Maximum safe concentration (MS<br><br><br><br>**Figure 1.2: Plasma drug concentration profiles** |

24

| | for conventional  tablet or capsule formulation ( - - - ) and a zero-order controlled-release formulation ( ___ ). MEC = Minimum Effective Concentration; MSC = Maximum Safe Concentration. |
|---|---|

| Benefit | Reasons |
|---|---|
| Patient comfort and compliance | 1. A reduction in dosing frequency enhances compliance.<br><br>2. The activity of the drug is extended throughout the night so that the patient can sleep undisturbed until morning.<br><br>3. Lessen the possibility of patient defaulting from the treatment by forgetting to take his medication. |
| Reduction in healthcare cost | 1. The total cost of therapy is lower.<br><br>2. Reduction in side effects reduces the expense in disease management.<br><br>3. Reduce the demand of the nursing stuff in the hospital. |

## 1.6   Disadvantages of Modified Release Dosage Forms

- The failure of modified release dosage form might lead to dose dumping. Dose dumping may be defined as the release of more than the usual fraction of drug or as the release of drug at a greater rate than the customary amount of drug per dosage interval, such that potentially adverse plasma levels may be reached (Dighe and Adams, 1988).

- On rare occasions, a prolonged action dosage form, like its non-prolonged action counterpart, becomes impeded in its transit through the GIT. This particularly troublesome for drugs which have high tendency to cause damage to the gastrointestinal mucosa (Roberts and Willium, 1975).

- Sustained release dosage form does not permit prompt termination of therapy when this is desired or required.

- They cost more per unit dose than regular dosage forms of the same drug.

- Patient to patient variation is a troublesome variable.

- Difficulties in manufacturing reproducibility.

- Total bioavailability may be lowered.

- The physician has less flexibility in adjusting dosage regimens.

- Patient would find it impossible to swallow if it is a bulky dosage form.

## 1.7 Factors Affecting Modified Release Dosage Forms

The overall factors (Robinson, 1978) that are considered in designing modified release dosage forms are given in the following table 1.2:

**Table 1.2: Factors consider in designing modified release dosage forms**

| Factors | Considerations |
|---|---|
| ▦ **Patient disease property** | ▪ Age and physiological state of patient<br>▪ Acute or chronic therapy required<br>▪ Pathology of disease<br>▪ Circadian changes in disease<br>▪ Ambulatory or bedridden<br>▪ Location of target area<br>▪ Route of drug administration<br>▪ Duration of intended drug action |
| ▦ **Drug properties** | ◆ Physicochemical<br>▪ Aqueous solubility<br>▪ Partition coefficient<br>▪ Charge<br>▪ pKa<br>▪ Molecular size<br>▪ Stability<br>◆ Biological<br>▪ Dose size<br>▪ Therapeutic index<br>▪ Fraction of dose absorbed<br>▪ Absorption rate constant<br>▪ Distribution<br>▪ Protein binding |
| ▦ **Drug properties** | ▪ Metabolism |

| | | ▪ Biological half-life |
| :--- | :--- | :--- |
| | | ◆ Physicochemical |
| | | ▪ Dissolution |
| | | ▪ Diffusion |
| | | ▪ Osmotic pump |
| | | ▪ Mechanical pump |
| **Delivery system** | | ▪ Ion exchange |
| **design** | | ▪ Combination of the above |
| | | ◆ Chemical modification |
| | | ▪ Analogs |
| | | ▪ Prodrugs |
| | | ◆ Biological |
| | | ▪ Enzyme inhibition |
| | | ▪ Increased biological half-life. |

## 1.8 Drugs Unsuitable For Modified Release Dosage Forms

- Drugs that are absorbed and excreted rapidly (having biological half life < 1hr.) e.g. Penicillin G.
- Drugs having long biological half life (>12 hrs.) e.g. Diazepam, Phenytoin.
- Drugs having low therapeutic indices e.g. Phenobarbital, Digitoxin.
- Rugs whose precision of dosage is important; e.g. anticoagulant and cardiac glycosides.

- Drugs that are not effectively absorbed from GIT. e.g. Riboflavin, Ferrous salts.
- Drugs having no clear advantage for sustained release formulation e.g. Griseofulvin
- Drugs whose large dose is required e.g. sulfonamides.

## 1.9    Methods of Sustaining Drug Action

Two general set of methods have been developed for implementation of practical extended release dosage form designs:

- Method based on modification of the physical and or chemical properties of the drugs.
- Method based on modification of the drug release rate characteristics of the dosage forms that affect the bioavailability of the drug.

A variety of techniques can be used to prepare oral extended release dosage forms, each technique offering some advantages and disadvantages. In some instances the principle of more than one technique is adopted in order to combine their maximize advantages & minimize their drawbacks. High doses of drugs administered in rapidly absorbed form have their own "Sustaining" effect relative to the elimination rate of lower doses. Nevertheless, it is not usually desirable to produce extended action by giving massive doses. There is a limit to the quantity of drug that can be administered at a time in massive dose safely to the patients. High doses can produce toxic reaction.

Considering this theme the basic methods of sustaining action are:

- Slowing or inhibiting inactivation of drugs producing pharmacological reaction.
- Slowing excretion or elimination of drug from the body.
- Changing physico-chemical properties of drug crystals.
- Controlling the release rate of drug from the dosage forms.

Different drug formulation methods used to obtain the desired drug release rate from extended release dosage form includes:

### 1.9.1 Increasing the Particle Size

Increasing the particle size causes decrease in surface area of the particles and decrease in release rate of the drug from the dosage form, as we know dissolution rate is directly proportional to the surface area exposed to the solvent.

### 1.9.2 Matrix System

Matrix system is that system, where the drug is dispersed in solid, which is less soluble or insoluble in fluid depot, making a continuous external phase of dispersion and effectively retards the passage of the drug from matrix system. The term matrix tablet describes a tablet in which the drug is applied in a skeleton of non-dissolving Material. It need simply direct compression of blended drugs and retarding additives to form tablets. It is one of the least complicated approaches to the manufacture of extended release dosage forms that consist of a drug dispersed in a polymer, the polymer playing the role of a matrix.

### 1.9.3 Coating System

The dosage form or individual particles are coated with materials that retard the drug release into the depot fluid and control the rate of availability of drug from dosage form. Drug release rate is dependent on the physico-chemical properties of the coating material.

### 1.9.4 Beads & Spheres

This kind of dosage form contains Beads or Spheres of drug, which are coated with material. The thickness of the coating material determines the times at which the drug will be released by diffusion through their pores.

### 1.9.5 Enteric Coated Beads in Capsules

The drug is incorporated in to beads or spheres of uniform size & uniformly coated with a suitable enteric materials, thus the rate of drug release depends on the stomach emptying rate of beads.

### 1.9.6 Repeat -action Tablet

Repeat-action tablets contain fraction of drug that dissolved or release of different times. They usually contain an immediate release fraction and other fractions periodically release the drug.

### 1.9.7 Mixed Release Granules

In this system two sets of granules are used one set contains immediate release component of drug and other set contains drug that are coated with dissolution retarding additives.

### 1.9.8 Erosion Core with Initial Dose

In this kind of extended product the drug is usually incorporated into tablet with insoluble materials such as high molecular weight Fats and Waxes. This is non-disintegrating tablets that maintain its geometric shape throughout the gastrointestinal tract. The initial also may be contained in Pan-Coated or Press Coated outer shell.The dissolution rate of drug from such tablet is directly proportional to the drug's solubility and tablet's surface area.

### 1.9.9 Erosion Core Only

The dosage form is formulated to contain only the extended release component. The primary purpose is to maintain a therapeutic consideration once therapy has been initiated.

### 1.9.10 The Ion Exchange Resins

The ion exchange method involves the administration of dosage form containing salt of drug complexes with an ion exchange resin that exchanges the drug for ions as it passes through the gastrointestinal tract. The ion exchange resins are water soluble cross linked polymer containing salt forming groups in repeating positions on the polymer chain. The drug is attached to the anionic or cationic groups and the drug release is retarded.

### 1.9.11 Complexation

The preparation of complex or salt of active drug that are highly soluble in the gastrointestinal fluid is the strategy used in this method of producing extended release products.

## 1.9.12 Micro encapsulation

Microcapsules are small particles that contain an active agent or core materials surrounded by a coating or shell. The release of the drug through the microencapsulated particles takes place by diffusion rather than by simple dissolution or disintegration. The drug diffuses through the wall of the microcapsules and dissolved in the gastrointestinal fluid. The microcapsule can be into capsules or tablet.

## 1.9.13 Osmotic Tablet

The osmotic tablet consists of core tablet and semi-permeable coating with a hole, produced by a laser beam. The drug exists through the hole due to the osmotic pressure, which occurs when the gastrointestinal fluid passes the semi-permeable membrane and reaches the core. The fluid dissolves the drug contained in the core and the osmotic pressure forces or pumps the drug solution out of the delivery orifice.

## 1.9.14 Encapsulated Slow Release Granules

In this type of dosage form the non-peril seeds are initially coated with adhesive and followed by powdered drug. The step is repeated until desired amount of drug has been applied. Then the granules are coated with mixture of solid hydroxylated lipids, which helps to sustain the release of active ingredient.

### 1.9.15 Gel forming Hydrocolloids

In this kind of dosage form the capsules are filled with dry mixture of drug and hydrocolloids. Upon dissolution the gastric fluid swells the outer most hydrocolloids to form gelatinous area, which acts as barrier and prevents the further penetration of gastric fluids. The gelatinous core erodes and new barrier layer forms. This process is continuous, releases the drug as each layer continues to erode and forms new layer. In particular, the interest awakened by matrix type deliveries is completely justified in view of their biopharmaceutical and pharmacokinetics advantages over the conventional dosage forms (Langer *et al.*, 1990). These are release systems for delay and control of the release of a drug that is dissolved or dispersed in a resistant support to disintegration. With the growing need for optimization therapy, matrix-systems providing programmable rate delivery other than the typical first-order delivery, are becoming more important (Qiu *et al.*, 1988).

### 1.10   Advancement in Methods of Sustaining Drug Action

Milo Gibaldi, Ph.D., dean of the University of Washington's School of Pharmacy in Seattle, writes in Biopharmaceutics and Clinical Pharmacokinetics:

> "The early history of the prolonged-release oral dosage form is probably best forgotten. Products were developed empirically, often with little rationale, and problems were common. Today, the situation has improved; many of the available products are well-designed drug delivery systems and have a defined

therapeutic goal. In some cases, the prolonged-release dosage form is the most important and most frequently used form of the drug."

In recent years, there have been numerous developments in polymeric carriers and controlled release systems. Some commercially available devices have been described by Lonsdale and Nixon, *1982*. A few examples mentioned in the literature include:

- Drug contained by a polymer containing a Hydrophilic and / or Leachable Additive eg, A second polymer, surfactant or plasticizer, etc. (Lordi., 1987; Udeala and Aly, 1989; Gardner, 1983).
- Enteric Coatings ionize and dissolve at a suitable pH (Gregoriadis, 1977).
- Soluble polymers with covalently attached 'Pendant' Drug molecules (Poznansky and Juliano, 1984; Tomlinson and Davis, 1986).
- Films with the drug in a Polymer Matrix / Monolithic Devices (Singh *et al.,* 1988)
- The drug contained by the polymer that acts as a Reservoir Devices (Nakagami *et al.*, 1991).
- Polymeric colloidal particles or microencapsulates (Microspheres or Nanoparticles) in the form of reservoir and matrix devices (Giddings *et al.*, 1975).
- Devices where release rate is controlled dynamically, *eg*, the Osmotic Pump (Patrick and McGinity, 1997).

## 1.11 Monolithic Devices (Matrix Devices)

The most common devices for controlling the release of drugs are monolithic (matrix) devices. This is possibly because they are relatively easy to fabricate, compared to reservoir devices, and there is not the danger of an accidental high dosage that could result from the rupture of the membrane of a reservoir device. In such a device the active agent is present as dispersion within the polymer matrix, and they are typically formed by the compression of a polymer/drug mixture or by dissolution or melting. The dosage release properties of monolithic devices may be dependent upon the solubility of the drug in the polymer matrix or, in the case of porous matrixes, the solubility in the sink solution within the particle's pore network, and also the tortuosity of the network (to a greater extent than the permeability of the film), dependent on whether the drug is dispersed in the polymer or dissolved in the polymer. For low loadings of drug, (0 to 5% W/V) the drug will be released by a solution-diffusion mechanism (in the absence of pores). At higher loadings (5 to 10% W/V), the release mechanism will be complicated by the presence of cavities formed near the surface of the device, as the drug is lost: such cavities fill with fluid from the environment increasing the rate of release of the drug. Generally release of drug form matrices will occur by a mixture of diffusion and erosion mechanisms. The swelling behaviour of swellable matrices is mechanistically described by front positions. Front position in the matrix where the physical conditions sharply change (Bettini *et al.*, 1998).

### 1.11.1 Matrix Tablet System

The term matrix tablet describes a tablet in which the drug is applied in a skeleton of non dissolving material. It needs simply direct compression of blended drugs and retarding additives to form tablets. It is one of the least complicated approaches to the manufacture of extended/controlled release dosage forms, which consists of a drug dispersed in a polymer, the polymer playing the role of a matrix ( Fessi *et al.*, 1982;

Focher *et al.*,1984; Heller,1984; Armand *et al.*,1987). Alternatively retardant-drug blends may be granulated prior to compression. It was found that the choice of matrix material, amount of drug incorporated in the matrix additives, the hardness of the tablet, density variation and tablet shape could markedly affect the release rate of drug (Capan, 1989). Matrix systems are economical. Beyond the possibility of lower development costs and the use of conventional production methods, the ingredients normally used are cost-effective. Matrix controlled release tablets are relatively simple systems that are more forgiving of variations in ingredients, production methods and end-use conditions than coated controlled release tablets and other systems. This results in more uniform release profiles with a high resistance to drug dumping.

There may be different classes of retardant materials used to formulate matrix tablets which are given below in table 1.3:

**Table 1.3: Materials used as retardants in matrix tablets**

| Matrix characteristics | Material |
|---|---|
| Insoluble, Inert (Plastic matrix) | Polyethylene<br>Polyvinyl chloride<br>Ethyl cellulose<br>Methyl acrylate –methacrylic acid copolymer<br>Cellulose acetate<br>Vinyl acetate/vinyl chloride copolymer |

| | Carnauba wax |
|---|---|
| Insoluble, erodable (Fat-Wax matrix) | Bees wax |
| | Stearic acid |
| | Paraffin wax |
| | High molecular weight polyethylene glycols |
| | Guar Gum |
| | Triglycerides |
| Hydrophilic | Methyl cellulose |
| | Sodium carboxymethyl cellulose |
| | Hydroxy propyl methyl cellulose |
| | Sodium alginate |
| | Gelatin |
| Hydrogel | Poly vinyl alcohol |
| | Poly hydroxyl alkyl methacrylates |
| | Ethylene vinyl alcohol and their copolymers. |

Several other workers (Desai *et al*, 1965) have also reported that the rate of drug released from a matrix is affected by:

- Drug solubility
- The composition of the matrix
- $P^H$ of the dissolution fluid
- Shape
- External agitation
- Mass of the drug
- and the porosity of the matrix

More recently Potter *et al.* (1992) observed that the particle size of the drug and excipient as well as the drug loading of tablets exert a great deal of effect on the release behavior.

The matrix tablet, which incorporates the active ingredient in an inert material matrix, has been well known to act as an effective extended release medicament. Inert soluble polymers have been used as a basis for many marketed formulations. Tablets prepared from materials are designed to be created in intact and not break apart in the gastrointestinal tract. Tablets may be directly compressed from mixtures of drug and retardant polymer; however, if ethyl cellulose is used as a matrix former, a wet granulation process using ethanol can be employed. The rate-limiting step in liquid penetration into the matrix unless channeling (wetting) agents are included to promote permeation of the polymer matrix by water, which allows drug dissolution and diffusion from the channels created in the matrix. Waxes, lipids and related materials form matrices that control release through both pore diffusion and erosion. Release characteristics are therefore more sensitive to digestive composition than the totally insoluble polymer matrix. Total release of drug from wax-lipid matrices is not possible in the absence of additives; drug release is prolonged and linear. Apparent zero – order release can be obtained by addition of additives such as polyvinyl pyrrolidone or polyoxy ethylene lauryl ethers. In a study by Dakkuri *et al.,* (1978), 10% to 20% hydrophilic polymers effectively controlled release from carnauba wax / stearyl alcohol matrices of tripelennamine hydrochloride. The third group of matrix formers represents hydrophilic matrix. These matrix systems have been proven for over four decades. A hydrophilic matrix, controlled-release system is a dynamic one involving polymer wetting, polymer hydration, gel formation, swelling and polymer dissolution. At the same time, other soluble excipients or drugs will also wet, dissolve and diffuse out of the matrix while insoluble materials will be held in place until the surrounding polymer/excipient/drug complex eroded or dissolves away. The mechanisms that drug controls release in matrix tablets are dependent on many variables. The main principle is that the water-soluble polymer, present throughout the tablet, hydrates on the outer tablet surface to form a gel layer. Throughout the life of the ingested tablet, the rate of drug release is determined by diffusion (if soluble) through the gel and by the rate of tablet erosion. Drug bioavailability, which is initially depending on the drug – polymer ratio, may be modified by inclusion of diluents such as lactose in place of polymer in the formulations. High drug polymer ratios result in formulation from which drug release is controlled by attrition (Salmon and Doelker, 1980). HPMC is a dominant vehicle for oral controlled release matrix tablets. The importance of the diffusion layer for a swollen matrix was illustrated in a mathematical model (Ford *et al.,* 1989)

Hydrogel hydrates on contact with water and water-soluble drugs are released by diffusion out of the gelatinous layer or by polymer erosion of the gel, whereas poorly soluble drugs are released slowly by erosion. Generally their release rate modulation is achieved using different grades of polymers different types of polymers, soluble fillers (Ford *et al.,* 1989), or insoluble fillers (Rao *et al.,*1988).

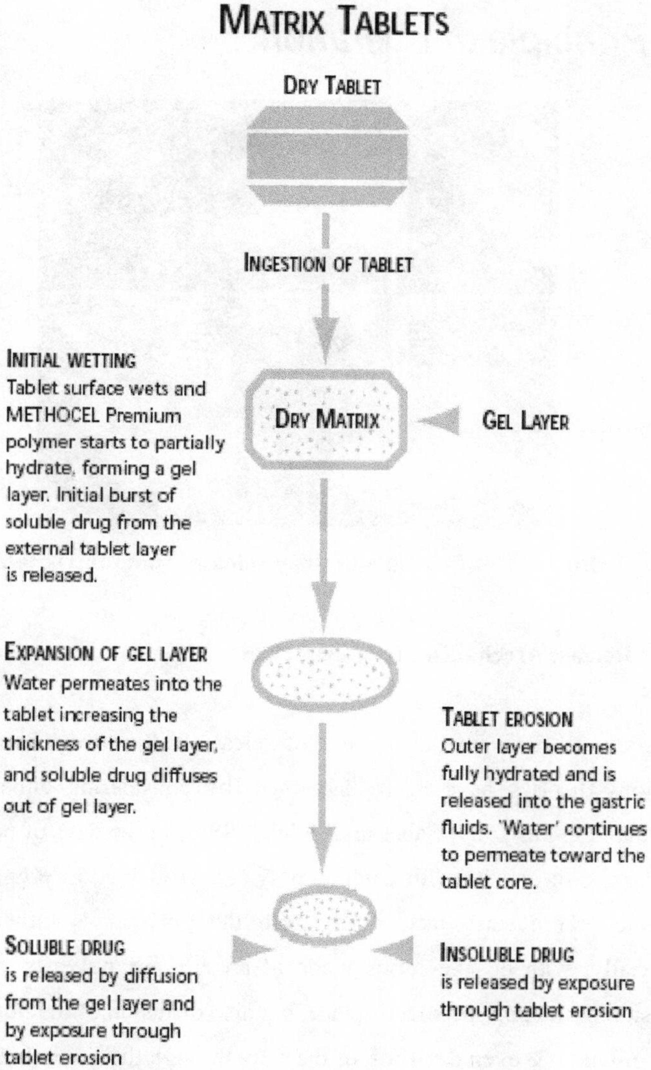

# MATRIX TABLETS

DRY TABLET

**INITIAL WETTING**
Tablet surface wets and
METHOCEL Premium
polymer starts to partially
hydrate, forming a gel
layer. Initial burst of
soluble drug from the
external tablet layer
is released.

INGESTION OF TABLET

DRY MATRIX ◄ GEL LAYER

**EXPANSION OF GEL LAYER**
Water permeates into the
tablet increasing the
thickness of the gel layer,
and soluble drug diffuses
out of gel layer.

**TABLET EROSION**
Outer layer becomes
fully hydrated and is
released into the gastric
fluids. 'Water' continues
to permeate toward the
tablet core.

**SOLUBLE DRUG**
is released by diffusion
from the gel layer and
by exposure through
tablet erosion

**INSOLUBLE DRUG**
is released by exposure
through tablet erosion

**Figure 1.3: Schematic diagram of drug release from matrix tablet**

# HYDROPHILIC MATRIX SYSTEMS
## *Principle of operation*

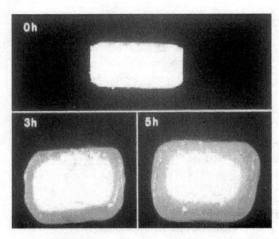

**Figure 1.4: Principle of drug release from matrix tablet**

### 1.12 Release Mechanism from Matrices

In order to describe the process of release of the drug from matrices, various theories have been elaborated, by considering either diffusion (Armand *et al.,* 1987; Saber and Pulak, 1988), in the case of non-erodible polymers, or erosion with erodible polymers (Bidah and Vergnaud, 1990). In fact, the release mechanism from the polymer is rather complex, specially, with dosage forms made of an erodible polymer, as not only erosion of the polymers takes place, but also diffusion of the liquid through the polymer & even diffusion of the drug through the liquid located within the polymer also takes place.

There are two other problems also of interest:

- When the solubility of the drug is low in the acid gastric fluid as well as the rate of dissolution & when it is necessary to help the drug dissolve in this liquid by provoking the extraction of the drug out of the dosage form. When the solubility is very low in the acid gastric liquid & rather high in the intestine where the pH is around 8.
- The polymer is rather complex, especially, with dosage forms made of an erodible polymer, as not only erosion of the polymer takesp lace, but also diffusion of the liquid through the polymer & even diffusion of the drug through the liquid located within the polymer (Liu. *et al.*, 1988)

There are four basic release systems for matrix formulations:

a) Inert Non-Bioerodible Matrix System

b) Bioerodible Matrix System

c) Swelling Controlled System

d) Magnetically Controlled System

In matrix system, the release is controlled by a combination of several physical processes. These includes:

- Permeation of the matrix by water
- Leaching (extraction or diffusion) of the drug from the matrix
- Erosion of the matrix material

Alternatively, the drug may dissolve in the matrix material and be related by diffusion through the matrix material or partitioned between the matrix and extracting fluids (Higuchi, 1963).

### 1.12.1 Inert Non - Bioerodible Matrix System

In inert non-bioerodible system, drug diffusion through the polymer matrix tablet is the rate limiting system. The system is schematically illustrated in fig 1.5.

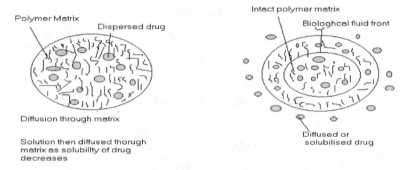

**Figure 1.5: Schematic diagram of an inert non-bioerodible matrix polymer drug delivery System.**

### 1.12.2 Bioerodible Matrix System

In bioerodible matrix system, the drug dispersed in a polymer and releases according to the rate of polymer bioerosion. The major advantage of bioerodible system is that the bioerodible polymer is eventually absorbed by the body. (Fig 1.6)

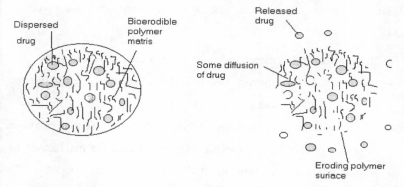

**Figure 1.6: Schematic diagram of a bioerodible polymeric drug delivery system**

Again it can be classified in two groups:

(a) bulk-eroding and

(b) surface-eroding biodegradable systems.

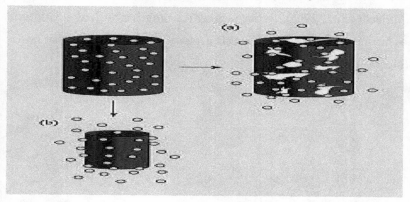

**Fig 1.7: Schematic diagram of a drug delivery from (a) bulk-eroding and (b) surface-eroding biodegradable systems.**

One of the major drawbacks of bioerodible systems are that as the release is eroded the surface area of the implant decreases. Bioerodiblep olymers release active drugs at a controlled rate via three major mechanism (Heller, 1984).

> Water-soluble polymers insolubilized by degradable cross-links
> Water insoluble polymers solubilized by hydrolysis, ionization or protonation of pendant side groups
> Water insoluble polymers solubilized by back-bone-chain cleavage in small water-soluble molecules. In most cases, the mechanism of solubilization is a combination of all three mechanisms.

### 1.12.3 Swelling Controlled System

In swelling controlled system, water penetrates into the matrices, the polymer particles swell modifying the matrix dimensions according to the loaded drug & polymer. The swelling of polymer particles arranged along a circumference involves an increase in the length of the circumference (Vandelli *et al.*, 1995). In this system, the drug is dissolved or dispersed within a polymer matrix tablet & is not able to diffuse through that matrix (Figure 1.7).

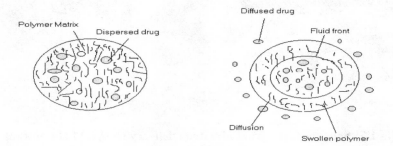

**Figure 1.8: Schematic diagram of swelling controlled system from matrix**

### 1.12.4 Magnetically Controlled System

In this system, drug & small magnetic beads are uniformly dispersed to viscous medium; drug is released in a fashion typical of diffusion controlled matrix system. However, upon exposure to an oscillating internal magnetic field, drug is released at a much higher rate. This is probably due to the compression of the polymer & dispersed magnets as illustrated in figure 1.8. (Langer and Peppas, 1981).

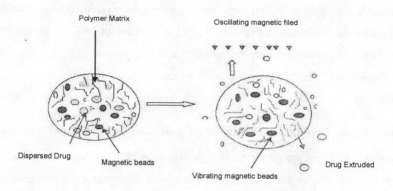

**Figure 1.9: Schematic diagram of a magnetically controlled polymeric drug deliver**

### 1.13 Classification of Rate Controlled Drug Delivery System

Based on the technical sophistication controlled release drug delivery systems that have recently been marketed or are under active development can be classified as follows:

    1) Rate Preprogrammed Drug Delivery Systems

2) Activation Modulated Drug Delivery Systems

3) Feedback Regulated Drug Delivery Systems

4) Site targeting Drug Delivery Systems

### 1.13.1 Rate-Preprogrammed Drug Delivery Systems

In this group of controlled- release drug delivery systems, the release of drug molecules from the delivery systems has been preprogrammed at specific rate profiles. This was accomplished by system design, which controls the molecular diffusion of drug molecules in and/ or across the barrier medium within or surrounding the delivery system. Fick's laws of diffusion are often followed. These systems can be further classified as follows:

### A) Polymer Membrane Permeation-Controlled Drug Delivery Systems

In this type of preprogrammed drug delivery systems, a drug formulation is totally or partially encapsulated within a drug reservoir compartment. Its drug release surface is covered by a rate controlling polymeric membrane having a specific permeability. The drug reservoir may exist in solid, suspension, or solution form. The polymeric membrane can be fabricated from a nonporous (homogeneous or heterogeneous) polymeric material or a micro porous (or semi-permeable) membrane. Injection molding, spray coating, capsulation, micro encapsulation, or other techniques accomplish the encapsulation of drug formulation inside the reservoir compartment. Different shapes and sizes of drug delivery systems can be fabricated.

### B) Polymer Matrix Diffusion – Controlled Drug Delivery Systems

In this type of preprogrammed drug delivery system, the drug reservoir is prepared by homogeneously dispersing drug particles in a rate –controlling polymer matrix fabricated from either a lipophilic or a hydrophilic polymer. The release of drug molecules from this type of controlled release drug delivery systems is controlled at a preprogrammed rate by controlling the loading dose, polymer solubility of the drug and its diffusivity in the polymer matrix.

## C) Micro reservoir Partition–Controlled Drug Delivery Systems

In this type of preprogrammed drug delivery systems the drug reservoir is fabricated by micro dispersion of an aqueous suspension of drug using a high-energy dispersion technique in a biocompatible polymer, such as silicone elastomers, to form a homogeneous dispersion of many discrete, unleachable, microscopic drug reservoirs. Different shapes and sizes of drug delivery devices can be fabricated from this micro reservoir drug delivery system by molding or extrusion.

## 1.13.2 Activation-Modulated Drug Delivery Systems

In this group of controlled release drug delivery systems, the release of drug molecules from the delivery systems is activated by some physical, chemical, or bio-chemical processes and/or facilitated by regulating the process applied or energy input. Based on the nature of the process applied or the type of energy used, these Cross-sectional view of the Syncro-Mate-C sub dermal implant fabricated from the microreservoir dissolution-controlled drug delivery system and the subcutaneous controlled release of

Norgestomet, a potent synthetic progestin, at a constant rate for up to 18 days (with 80% loading dose released).

The open ends on the implant do not affect the zero-order in vivo drug release profile activation - modulated drug delivery systems can be classified into the following categories:

**Physical means**

    A. Osmotic Pressure Activated Drug Delivery Systems

    B. Hydrodynamic Pressure Activated Drug Delivery Systems

    C. Vapor Pressure Activated Drug Delivery Systems

    D. Mechanically Activated Drug Delivery Systems

    E. Magnetically Activated Drug Delivery Systems

    F. Sonophoresis Activated Drug Delivery Systems

    G. Iontophoresis Activated Drug Delivery Systems

    H. Hydration Activated Drug Delivery Systems

**Chemical means**

    I. pH Activated Drug Delivery Systems

    J. Ion Activated Drug Delivery Systems

    K. Hydrolysis activated Drug Delivery Systems

**Biochemical means**

    L. Enzyme activated drug delivery systems

Several systems have been successfully developed and applied clinically to the controlled delivery of pharmaceuticals. These are outlined and discussed in a short in the following:

## A. Osmotic pressure-Activated Drug Delivery Systems

This type of activation-controlled drug delivery system depends on osmotic pressure to activate the release of drug. In this system the drug reservoir, which can be either a solution or a solid formulation, is contained within a semi-permeable housing with controlled 2water permeability. The drug is activated to release in solution from at a constant rate through a special delivery orifice. Controlling the gradient of osmotic pressure modulates the rate of drug release.

## B. Hydrodynamic Pressure-Activated Drug Delivery Systems

A hydrodynamic pressure-activated drug delivery system can be fabricated by enclosing a collapsible, impermeable container, which contains a liquid drug formulation to form a drug reservoir compartment, inside a rigid shape-retaining house. Osmotic pressure-activated drug delivery system and the effect of increased osmotic pressure in the delivery system on the release profiles of Phenyl propanolamine HCl from the Acutrim tablet at intestinal condition.

## C. Vapor Pressure-Activated Drug Delivery Systems

Vapor pressure has also been discovered as a potential energy source to activate the delivery of therapeutic agents. In this type of drug delivery system the drug reservoir, which also exists as a solution formulation, is contained inside the infusion compartment. It is physically separated from the pumping compartment by a freely movable partition. The pumping compartment contains a fluorocarbon fluid that vaporizes at body temperature at the implantation site and creates vapor pressure. Under the vapor pressure created the partition moves upward.

## D. Mechanically Activated Drug Delivery Systems

In this type of activation-controlled drug delivery system the drug reservoir is a solution formulation retained in a container equipped with a mechanically activated pumping system. A measured dose of drug formulation is reproducibly delivered into a body cavity, for example the nose, through the spray head upon manual activation of the drug delivery pumping system. The volume of solution delivered is controllable, as small as 10-100μl, and is independent of the force and duration of activation applied as well as the solution volume in the container. A typical example of this type of rate-controlled drug delivery system is the development of a metered-dose of buselin, a synthetic analog of luteinizing hormone releasing hormone (LHRH) and insulin

## E. Magnetically Activated Drug Delivery Systems

In this type o activation-controlled drug delivery system the drug reservoir is a dispersion of peptide or protein powders in a polymer matrix from which macromolecular drug can be improved by incorporating an electromagnetically triggered vibration mechanism into the polymeric delivery device. The hemispherical magnetic delivery device produced has been used to deliver protein drugs, such as bovine serum albumin, at a low basal rate, by a simple diffusion process under nontriggering conditions. As the magnet is activated to vibrate by an external electromagnetic field, the drug molecules are delivered at a much higher rate.

## F. Sonophoresis – Activated Drug Delivery System

This type of activation-controlled drug delivery systems utilizes ultrasonic energy to activate (or trigger) the delivery of drugs from a polymeric drug delivery device. The system can be fabricated from either a nondegradable polymer, such as ethylene-vinyl acetate copolymer, or a bioerodible polymer, such as poly [bis (p-carboxyphenoxy) alkane anhydride]. The potential application of sonophoresis (or phonophoresis) to regulate the delivery of drugs was recently reviewed.

## G. Iontophoresis – Activated Drug Delivery Systems

This type of activation controlled drug delivery systems uses electrical current to activate and to modulate the diffusion of a charged drug molecule across a biological membrane, like the skin, in a manner similar to passive diffusion under a concentration gradient, but at a much-facilitated rate.

## H. Hydration-Activated Drug Delivery Systems

This type of activation controlled drug delivery systems depends on the hydration induced swelling process to activate the release of drug. In this system the drug reservoir is homogeneously dispersed in a swell able polymer matrix fabricated from a hydrophilic polymer. The release of drug is controlled by the rate of swelling of the polymer matrix.

## I. pH- Activated Drug Delivery Systems

This type of activation-controlled drug delivery system permits targeting the delivery of a drug only on the region with a selected pH range. It is fabricated by coating the drug-containing core with a pH sensitive polymer combination. For instance, a gastric fluid-labile drug is protected by encapsulating it inside a polymer membrane that resists the degradative action of gastric pH, such as the combination of ethyl cellulose and hydroxyl methylcellulose phthalate.

## J. Ion-Activated Drug Delivery Systems

In addition to the iontophoresis activated drug delivery system just discussed, an ionic or a charged drug can be delivered by an ion-activated drug delivery system. Such a system is prepared by first complexing an ionic drug with an ion-exchange resin containing a suitable counter ion, for example, by forming a complex between a cationic drug with a resin having a $SO_3$ group or between an anionic drug with a resin having a $N(CH_3)^+_3$ Group.

## K. Hydrolysis-Activated Drug Delivery Systems

This type of activation-controlled drug delivery system depends on the hydrolysis process to activate the release of drug molecules. In this system the drug reservoir is either encapsulated in microcapsules or homogeneously dispersed in micro spheres or nanoparticles for injection. It can also be fabricated as an implantable device. All these systems are prepared from a bioerodible or biodegradable polymer, such as co (Lactic-glycolic) polymer, pol (orthoester), or poly (anhydride). The release of a drug from the polymer matrix is activated by the hydrolysis-induced degradation of polymer chains and controlled by the rate of polymer degradation. A typical example of a hydrolysis activated drug delivery system is the development of LHRH-releasing biodegradable subdermal implant, which is designed to delivery goserelin, a synthetic LHRH analog, for once-a month treatment of prostate carcinoma.

## M. Enzyme-Activated Drug Delivery Systems

This type of activation controlled drug delivery system depends on the enzymatic process to activate the release of drug. In this system the drug reservoir is either physically entrapped in micro spheres or chemically bound to polymer chains from biopolymers, such as albumins or polypeptides. The release of drugs is activated by the enzymatic hydrolysis of the biopolymers by a specific enzyme in the target tissue. A typical example of this enzyme activated drug delivery system is the development of albumin micro spheres that release 5-fluorouracil in a controlled manner by protease activated biodegradation.

## 1.13.3 Feedback-Regulated Drug Delivery Systems

In this group of controlled release drug delivery systems the release of drug molecules from the delivery systems is activated by a triggering agent, such as a biochemical substance, in the body and also regulated by its concentration via some feedback mechanisms. The rate of drug release is then controlled by the Amino acid sequence of goserelin, a synthetic LHRH, and the effect of subcutaneous controlled release of goserelin from the biodegradable poly (lactide-glycolide) sub dermal implant on the serum levels of LH and testosterone.

## A. Bioerosion-Regulated Drug Delivery System

Heller and Trescony applied the feedback- regulated drug delivery concept to the development of a bioerosion regulated drug delivery system. The system consisted of drug dispersed bioerodible matrix fabricated from poly (vinyl methyl ether) half-ester, which was coated with a layer of immobilized urease. In a solution with near neutral pH, the polymer only erodes very slowly. In the presence of urea, urease at the surface of drug delivery system metabolizes urea to form a Cross sectional view of a bioerosion regulated hydrocortisone delivery system, a feedback regulated drug delivery system, showing the drug dispersed monolithic bioerodible polymer matrix with surface immobilized ureases.

## B. Bioresponsive Drug Delivery Systems

The feedback regulated drug delivery concept has also been applied to the development of a bioresponsive drug delivery system. In this system the drug reservoir is contained in a device enclosed by a bioresponsive polymeric membrane whose drug permeability is controlled by the concentration of a biochemical agent in the tissue where the system is located.

## C. Self – Regulating Drug Delivery Systems

In this system the drug reservoir is a drug complex encapsulated within a semi permeable polymeric membrane. The release of the drug from the delivery system is activated by the membrane permeation of a biochemical agent from the tissue in which the system is located.

### 1.13.4 Site – targeted Drug Delivery Systems

Delivery of a drug to a target tissue that needs medication is known to be a complex process consisting of multiple steps of diffusion and partitioning. Ideally, the path of drug transport should also be under control. Then, the ultimate goal of optimal treatment with maximal safety can be reached. Unfortunately, this ideal site targeting controlled release drug delivery system is only in the conceptual stage. Its construction remains a largely unresolved, challenging task for the biomedical and pharmaceutical sciences.

### 1.14 Types of retardant materials used to formulate matrix tablets

There may be three types of retardant materials used to formulate matrix tablets.

Such as –

i)   Polymers forming insoluble or skeleton matrices constitute the first category of retarding materials, also classed as plastic matrix systems

ii)  The second class represents hydrophobic and water- insoluble materials.

iii) While the third group includes polymers those form hydrophilic matrices.

List of three types of polymers which are commonly used in sustain release dosage form that shown in Table1.4:

**Table 1.4 List of Hydrophilic, Hydrophobic & Plastic Polymers which are commonly used in sustain release dosage form (Fambri *et.al.*, 1996)**

| Sl No | Hydrophilic Polymer | Hydrophobic Polymer | Plastic Polymer |
|-------|---------------------|---------------------|-----------------|
| 1. | Alginic Acid | Avicel PH 101 | Eudragit RL PO |
| 2. | Cabomer 940 | Avicel PH 102 | Eudragit RL 100 |
| 3. | Gelatin | Bees wax | Eudragit RS PO |
| 4. | Guar Gum | Cellulose acetate (CAP) | Eudragit RL 100 |
| 5. | Hydroxypropyl methyl cellulose -Methocel K15M | Carnauba wax | Eudragit RL 100 |
| 6. | Hydroxypropyl methyl cellulose –Methocel K100 LVCR | Cetyl alcohol | Kollidon SR |
| 7. | Kollicoat IR 0000 | Ethyl cellulose | |
| 8. | Ludipress LCE | Glyceyl monostearate (GMS) | |
| 9. | Ludipress | Hydroxy propyl methyl cellulose phthalate 40 cst (HPMCP 40 cst) | |
| 10. | Modified starch | Hydroxy propyl methyl | |

| 12. | Polyethylene glycol 4000(PEG 4000) | Stearic alcohol |
| --- | --- | --- |
| 13. | Polyethylene glycol 6000(PEG 6000) | |
| 14. | Polyethylene glycol 20,000 (PEG 20,000) | |
| 15. | Polyvinyl alcohol | |
| 16. | Sodium carboxy methyl cellulose 8000cps (NaCMC 8000 cps ) | |
| 17. | Sodium carboxy methyl cellulose 10000 cps (NaCMC 10000 cps ) | |
| 18. | Sodium Alginate | |

## 1.15 The "Ideal" polymer for drug delivery

Various as well as natural polymers have been examined in drug delivery applications. If the polymer matrix does not degrade inside the body, then it has to be surgically removed after it is depleted of the drug. Hence to avoid the costs as well as risks associated with multiple surgeries, the polymer used should be biologically degradable. Thus for a polymer to be used as a drug delivery matrix, it has to satisfy the following criteria:

I. It has to be biocompatible and degradable (i.e. it should degrade *in vivo* to smaller fragment which can then be excreted from the body.)

II. The degradation products should he nontoxic and should not create an inflammatory response.

59

III.    Degradation should occur within a reasonable period of time as required by the application.

## 1.16  Role of Polymeric drug Delivery

There has been a rapid growth in recent years in the area of drug discovery, facilitated by novel technologies such as combinatorial chemistry and high-throughput screening. These novel approaches have led to drugs that are generally more potent and have poorer solubility than drugs developed from traditional approaches of medicinal chemistry (Lipinsky and Paronen, 1998). The development of these complex drugs has resulted in a more urgent focus on developing novel techniques, to deliver these drugs more effectively and efficiently.

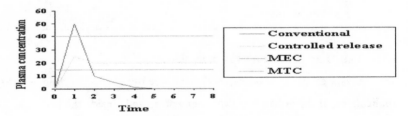

**Figure 1.10: Conventional and Ideal drug release profiles.**

It has been observed from above figure that the conventional oral and intravenous routes of drug administration do not provide ideal pharmacokinetic profiles especially for drugs, which display high toxicity and/or narrow therapeutic windows. For such drugs the ideal pharmacokinetic profile will be one wherein the drug concentration reached therapeutic levels without exceeding the maximum tolerable dose and maintains these concentrations for extended periods of time till the desired therapeutic effect is reached. One of the ways such a profile can be achieved in an ideal case scenario would be by encapsulating the drug in a polymer matrix. The technology of polymeric drug delivery has been studied in details over the past 30 years and numerous excellent reviews are available (Gombotz and Pettie, 1995; Sinha and Khosla, 1998; Langer, 1998). The three key advantages that polymeric drug delivery products can offer are:

1. **Localized delivery of drug:** The product can be implanted directly at the site where drug action is needed and hence systemic exposure of the drug can be reduced. This becomes especially important for toxic drugs that are related to various systemic side effects (such as the chemotherapeutic drugs).

2. **Extended delivery of drugs:** The drug encapsulated is released over extended periods and hence eliminates the need for multiple injections. This feature can improve patient compliance especially for drugs for chronic indications, requiring frequent injections (such as for deficiency of certain proteins).

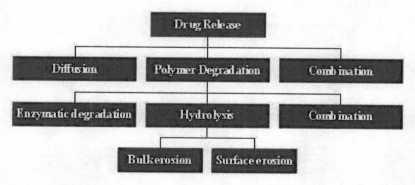

**Figure 1.11: Possible drug release mechanisms for polymeric drug delivery**

3. **Stabilization of the drug:** The polymer can protect the drug from the physiological environment and hence improve its stability *in vivo*. This particular feature makes this technology attractive for the delivery of labile drugs such as proteins.

Figure 1.11 shows that the drug will be released over time either by diffusion out of the polymer matrix or by degradation of the polymer backbone. The continuous release of drugs from the polymer matrix could occur either by diffusion of the drug from the polymer matrix, or by the erosion of the polymer (due to degradation) or by a combination of the two mechanisms. Several reviews have been presented on the mechanisms and the mathematical aspects of release of drugs from polymer matrices (Batycky *et al.*, 1997; Brazel *et al.*, 2000; Comets and Sannet, 2000). For a given drug, the release kinetics from the polymer matrix are governed predominantly by three factors:

  a) The polymer type,

  b) Polymer morphology and

  c) The excipients present in the system.

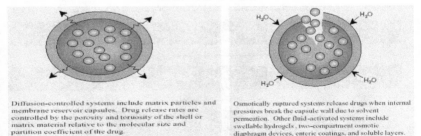

Diffusion-controlled systems include matrix particles and membrane reservoir capsules. Drug release rates are controlled by the porosity and tortuosity of the shell or matrix material relative to the molecular size and partition coefficient of the drug.

Osmotically ruptured systems release drugs when internal pressures break the capsule wall due to solvent permeation. Other fluid-activated systems include swellable hydrogels, two-compartment osmotic diaphragm devices, enteric coatings, and soluble layers.

**Figure 1.12: Mechanism of Polymeric Drug Delivery (Controlled Release Methods)**

In Figure 1.13, a polymer and active agent have been mixed to form a homogeneous system, also referred to as a matrix system. Diffusion occurs when the drug passes from the polymer matrix into the external environment. As the release continues, its rate normally decreases with this type of system, since the active agent has a progressively longer distance to travel and therefore requires a longer diffusion time to release.

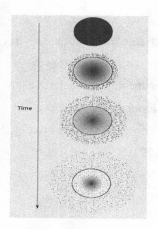

**Figure 1.13: Drug delivery from a typical matrix.**

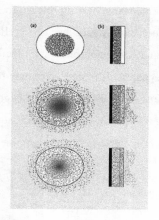

**Figure 1.14: Drug delivery from typical reservoir devices**

(a) Implantable or oral systems,

(b) Transdermal systems.

For the reservoir systems shown in Figure 1.13, the drug delivery rate can remain fairly constant. In this design, a reservoir - whether solid drug, dilute solution, or highly concentrated drug solution within a polymer matrix - is surrounded by a film or membrane of a rate-controlling material. The only structure effectively limiting the release of the drug is the polymer layer surrounding the reservoir.

## 1.17 Mathematical Models of Release Mechanisms from Matrices

### 1.17.1 Release from Soluble Retardants

The Mechanisms of drug release from various polymeric matrix systems have been extensively discussed (Higuchi, 1963; Roseman and Cardinelli, 1980). The diffusion of drug molecules to & from the matrix across the hydrodynamic diffusion layer may be treated as one-dimensional diffusion to a plane surface (Perkin and Beageal, 1971). From earlier theoretical treatments, the following general equations describing the release of drug from a polymeric matrix are obtained (Chien, 1992).

$$d_s^2 + \frac{2D_s d_d d_s}{KD_s} = \frac{4CpD_s t}{(2A - Cs)} \ldots\ldots\ldots(Eq.1)$$

$$Q = (A - C_s/2)\, d_S \ldots\ldots\ldots\ldots\ldots\ldots\ldots\ldots(Eq.2)$$

Where $d_s$ and $d_d$ are the thicknesses of the depletion zone and the hydrodynamic diffusion layer, respectively; $D_d$ & $D_s$ are the diffusivities of drug in the matrix phase & the solution phase respectively; A is the total amount of solid drug impregnated per unit volume of polymeric matrix; $C_p$ and $C_s$ are the drug solubility in the polymer and in the solution respectively; K is the partition-co-efficient of the drug species from the matrix phase to the elution medium; Q is the amount of drug released per unit surface area of devices ; and t is time :

For a matrix controlled process:

$$d_s^2 \ggg \frac{2D_s d_d d_s}{KD_s} \quad \ldots\ldots\ldots\ldots\ldots\ldots\ldots\ldots\text{(Eq.3)}$$

Then equation (1) is reduced to:

$$D_s^2 = \frac{4CpD_s t}{(2A - Cs)} \quad \ldots\ldots\ldots\ldots\ldots\ldots\ldots\ldots\ldots\ldots\ldots\text{(Eq .4)}$$

Or , $\quad d_s = 2[\dfrac{CpDst}{2A - Cs}]^{1\backslash 2} \quad \ldots\ldots\ldots\ldots\ldots\ldots\ldots\text{(Eq .5)}$

Substituting eq (5) for ds in eq (2) results in:

$$Q = \sqrt{} \ \{d_s\,(2a - c_s)\,c_p t \ \} \quad \ldots\ldots\ldots\ldots\ldots\ldots\text{(Eq .6)}$$

Ordinarily, a $\gg c_s$ and equation (6) is reduced to:

$$Q = [2ad_s c_p t]^{-1\backslash 2} \quad \ldots\ldots\ldots\ldots\ldots\ldots\ldots\ldots\ldots\ldots\ldots\ldots\text{(Eq .7)}$$

A, Ds & Cp are constants for a particular system and when $\sqrt{}\,2ADsC_p$ replaced by $k_1$, the equation (7) reduces to simplified equation (8),

$$Q = k\sqrt{}\ t \quad \ldots\ldots\ldots\ldots\ldots\ldots\ldots\ldots\ldots\text{(Eq. 8)}$$

Equation (8) includes that the amount of drug released is proportional to the square root of time, which is well known as Higuchi equation.

### 1.17.2: Release from Insoluble Retardants

The equation describing drug release from the planar surface of an insoluble matrix is as follows (Higuchi, 1963):

$$Q = [ (DEC_S/T)(2A - EC_S)t ]^{1\backslash2} \quad ...................(Eq .9)$$

Where Q is the amount of drug released per unit surface after time t. D is the diffusion co-efficient of the drug in the elution medium, T is the tortuosity of the matrix, E is the porosity of the matrices. Cs is the solubility of the drug in the elution medium & A is the initial loading does of drug in the matrix.

The expression both from equation (6) & (9) were derived as summing a linear diffusion gradient as diagrammed in (Figure 1.14) Drug release is triggered by penetration of eluting media into the matrix, dissolving drug, thereby creating channels through which diffusion takes place (Figure 1.17.2). The depletion zone gradually extends into the core of matrix. A high tortuosity means that the effective average diffusion path is large. The porosity term takes place into account the space available for drug dissolution; an increased porosity results in increased drug release (Figure 1.17.2). Both porosity & tortuosity are functions of the amount of dispersed drug, the physico-chemical properties of the matrix & the dispersion characteristics of the drug in the matrix (Lordi, 1987).

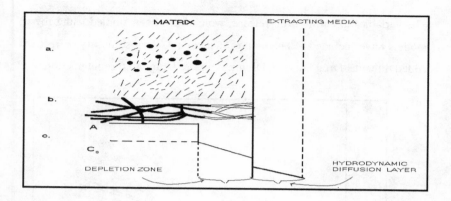

**Figure 1.15: Embedded matrix concept as a mechanism of controlled release in extended release dosage form design. Network model (a): drug is insoluble in the retardant material. Dispersion model b): drug is soluble in the retardant material. Diffusion profile (c) Characterizes drug release from a matrix system.**

### 1.17. 3 Drug Release of Low Solubility in Elution

If the drug has low solubility in the elution media, partition control dominates & the release is zero-order, that is:

$$Q = KDC_s \, t / h \quad ............................(Eq .10)$$

Where, k is the partition co-efficient ($k = c_s/c_p$). Cp is the solubility in the matrix phase, & H is the thickness of the hydrodynamic diffusion layer.

The variables affecting drug release, which have been studied using these models have included – The nature of retardant, drug solubility, Effect of added diluents, Drug loading, Drug mixture & Drug mixture interaction.

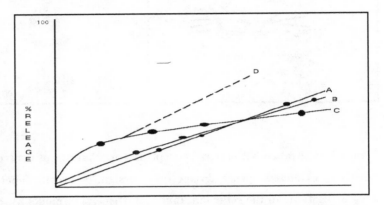

**Figure 1.16: Drug-release profile characteristic of different dosage form models representing embedded matrix systems. A, Zero - order model. B, First - order model . C, Diffusion model.  D, Diffusion model with erosion.**

**1.18 Biexponential Model**

In swellable matrices, the release of the drug is controlled by one or more of the following processes:

- The diffusion of water into the matrix;
- The swelling due to the hydration of the matrix or the relaxation of the polymer chains (often referred to as case II transport);
- Diffusion of the drug through the swollen matrix and through the existing pores, in any, and
- The dissolution or erosion of the matrices.

The overall profile depends on which process of combination of processes dominant the release. A simple expression that may be used to to model these processes is that suggested by Beren and Hophenberg., 1978.

$$M_t / M_\alpha = K_1 t + K_2 t^{1/2} \quad \text{--------------(Eq.11)}$$

Where, $M_t / M_\alpha$ is the fraction released in time $t$, and $K_1$ & $K_2$ are constants describing the constant rate process (erosion) and diffusion controlled release mechanisms, respectively.

The advantages of this expression in that it separates the effects of two simultaneous Processes and that $K_1$ and $K_2$ have a meaningful physical interpretation. The example - (Eq.11) includes $k_1$, the effect of polymer relaxation and the so called case- II transport. The phenomenon is generally attributed to structrural changes induced in the polymer by the penetrant (Peterlin, 1979, 1980) which cause the polymer to swell. If this process is the rate limiting step, the release of drug from the matrix will be zero order and is called relaxation controlled, swelling- controlled or case II transport process (Korsmeyer *et al., 1983;* Peppas *et al., 1986).* However, *Hopenberg (1976)* suggested that the most simple relaxation process might be dissolution of the polymer. Therefore, $k_1$ can be associated with the dissolution as well as relaxation of polymer chains. *Lee* (1980) formulated a drug release model from erodible matrices which has dissolution contribution (but no swelling component) and came to the same empirical form as equation (11).

It can be seen from equation (11), that the release can be approximated by t ½ ($k_2$), zero order ($k_1$) or mixed kinetics ($k_2$ and $k_1$) if it is controlled by diffusion, case II transport (or dissolution of the polymer) and a mixture of the two (anomalous or non-Fickian transport), respectively. In addition, the simple power law expression shown in equation (11) may be used to correlate and evaluate release data (Langer *et al.*, 1981).

$$M_t / M_\alpha = K^n \text{---------------- (Eq.12)}$$

Where k is a constant and n is a release exponent, indicative of the mechanism of drug release. The drug release were plotted in Korsmeyer et al's equation (Eq. 13) as log cumulative percent of drug release vs log time and the exponent n was calculated through the slope of the straight line.

$$M_t / M_\alpha = Kt^n \text{----------------(Eq. 13)}$$

Where $M_t / M_\alpha$ is the fractional solute release, t is the release time, K is a kinetic constant and n is an exponent that characterizes the mechanism of release of tracers.

Table 1.5 shows an analysis of diffusional release mechanism obtained by varying the n values (Langer *et al.*, 1981). The n values used for analysis of the drug release mechanism from the tablets were determined from log ($M_t / M_\alpha$) vs log (t) plots.

**Table 1.5:** Geometric dependence of diffusional exponent (n) and variation of n values with mechanism of diffusion

| Diffusional exponent (n) | | | Mechanism of transport |
| Cylinder | Sphere | Slab | |
|---|---|---|---|
| < 0.45 or 0.45 | < 0.43 or 0.43 | < 0.50 or 0.5 | Fickian (case I) diffusion |
| >0.45 or < 0.89 | >0.43 and <0.85 | >0.5 and <1.0 | Anomalous / non – Fickian transport |
| 0.89 | 0.85 | 1.0 | Case II / Zero order transport |
| >0.89 | >0.85 | >1.0 | Super Case II transport |

## 1.19 Bioequivalence Study

Bioequivalence testing is considered as a surrogate for clinical evaluation of the therapeutic equivalence of drug products based on the fundamental bioequivalence assumption that when two drug products (for example, a brand-name drug and its generic copy) are equivalent in bioavailability, they will reach the same therapeutic effect. Bioavailability for in vivo bioequivalence studies is usually assessed through the measures of the rate and extent to which the drug product is absorbed into the bloodstream of human subjects. For some locally acting drug products such as nasal aerosols (for example, metered-dose inhalers) and nasal sprays (for example, metered-dose spray pumps) that are not intended to be absorbed into the bloodstream, bioavailability may be assessed by measurements intended to reflect the rate and extent to which the active ingredient or active moiety becomes available at the site of action. For these local delivery drug products, the U.S. Food and Drug Administration (FDA)

71

indicates that bioequivalence may be assessed, with suitable justification, by in vitro bioequivalence studies alone. It is recognized that in vitro methods are less variable, easier to control, and more likely to detect differences between products (Saudi Food and Drug Authority, 2005).

### *Bioavailability*

Bioavailability means the rate and extent to which the active drug substance or therapeutic moiety is absorbed from a pharmaceutical dosage form and becomes available at the site of action. For drugs intended to exhibit a systemic therapeutic effect, bioavailability can be more simply understood as the rate and extent to which a substance or its therapeutic moiety is delivered from a pharmaceutical dosage form into the general circulation. Indeed, in the case of such drugs, the substance in the general circulation is in exchange with the substance at the site of action.

### *Bioequivalence*

Is defined as the absence of a significant difference in the rate and extent to which the active ingredient or active moiety in pharmaceutical equivalents or pharmaceutical alternatives becomes available at the site of drug action when administered at the same molar dose under similar conditions in an appropriately designed study.

For any type of bioequivalence study referenced is used. A reference product is a pharmaceutical product with which the new product is intended to be interchangeable in clinical practice. The reference product would normally be the innovator product for which efficacy, safety and quality have been established. Generally, the innovator pharmaceutical product is that which was authorized for marketing (normally as a patented drug) on the basis of documentation of efficacy, safety and quality (according to contemporary requirements). In the case of drugs, which have been available for many years, it may not be possible to identify an innovator pharmaceutical product. When the innovator product is not available the product which is the market leader may be used as a reference product, provided that it has been authorized for marketing and its efficacy, safety and quality have been established and documented.

Pharmaceutically equivalent multi-source pharmaceutical products must be shown to be therapeutically equivalent to one another in order to be considered interchangeable. Several test methods are available to assess equivalence, including:

(A) Comparative bioavailability (bioequivalence) studies in humans in which the active drug substance or one or more metabolites are measured in an accessible biologic fluid such as plasma, blood or urine.

(B)  Comparative pharmacodynamic studies in humans.

(C)  Comparative clinical trials.

(D) In-Vitro Studies.

Acceptance of any test procedure in the documentation of equivalence between two pharmaceutical products by the drug regulatory authority depends on many factors, including characteristics of the active drug substance and the drug product. Where a drug produces meaningful concentrations in an accessible biological fluid, such as plasma, comparative bioavailability (bioequivalence) studies are preferred. Where a

73

drug does not produce measurable concentrations in an accessible biological fluid, comparative clinical trials or pharmacodynamic studies may be necessary to document equivalence. In vitro testing, preferably based on a documented in vitro / in vivo correlation, may sometimes provide same indication of equivalence between two pharmaceutical products.

## 1.19.1 Bioequivalance studies in Human bassed on Pharmakokinetics Measures

The definition of bioequivalence expressed in terms of rate and extent of absorption of the active ingredient or moiety to the site of action, emphasize the use of pharmacokinetic measures in an accessible biological matrix such as blood, plasma, or serum and/or urine to indicate the release of the drug substance from the drug product into the systemic circulation. This approach resets on the understanding that measuring the active moiety or ingredient at the site of action is generally not possible and, furthermore, that some relationship exists between the efficacy/safety and concentration of the active moiety and / or its important metabolite(s) in the systemic circulation. Bioequivalence studies are designed to compare the in vivo performance of a test pharmaceutical product (multi-source) compared to a reference pharmaceutical product. A common design for a bioequivalence study involves administration of the test and reference products on two occasions to volunteer subjects, with each administration separated by a washout period. The washout period is chosen to ensure that drug given in one treatment is entirely eliminated prior to administration of the next treatment. Just prior to administration, and for a suitable period afterwards, blood and/or urine samples are collected and assayed for the concentration of the drug substance and/or one or more metabolites. The rise and fall of these concentrations over time in each subject in the study provide an estimate of how the drug substance is released from the test and reference products and absorbed into the body. To allow comparisons between the two products, these blood (to include plasma or serum) and/ or urine concentration time curves are used to calculate certain pharmacokinetic parameters of interest. These parameters are calculated for each subject in the study and the resulting values are compared statistically.

Bioequivalence of systemically absorbed drugs are assessed using pharmacokinetic (bioavailability) endpoints provided the drug concentrations in the biological matrix can be accurately measured. However, for nonabsorbable drug products and those that are intended for topical administration, bioequivalence is assessed by evaluating pharmacodynamic or clinical endpoints or by in vitro test methods. Some examples are : Topical dermatologic corticosteroids are evaluated by a " Skin Blanching Test " (vasoconstrictor assay), topical anti-infective drugs by clinical tests comparing efficacy profiles, metered dose inhalers by pulmonary function tests, and cholesterol lowering resin powder by in vitro binding tests.

## 1.19.2 Pharmacodynamic Studies

Studies in healthy volunteers or patients using pharmacodynamic measurements may be used for establishing equivalence between two pharmaceutical products. These studies may become necessary if quantitative analysis of the drug and/or metabolite(s) in plasma or urine cannot be made with sufficient accuracy and sensitivity. Furthermore, pharmacodynamic studies in humans are required if measurements of drug concentrations cannot be used as surrogate endpoints for the demonstration of efficacy and safety of the particular pharmaceutical product e.g., for topical products without intended absorption of the drug into the systemic circulation. If pharmacodynamic studies are to be used they must be performed as rigorously as bioequivalence studies, and the principles of Good Clinical Practice (GCP) must be followed.

### 1.19.3 Clinical Studies

In several instances, plasma concentration time-profile data are not suitable to assess bioequivalence between two formulations. Whereas in some of the cases pharmacodynamic studies can be an appropriate tool for establishing equivalence, in other instances this type of study cannot be performed because of lack of meaningful pharmacodynamic parameters which can be measured and a comparative clinical trial has to be performed in order to demonstrate equivalence between two formulations. However, if a clinical study is considered as being undertaken to prove equivalence, the same statistical principles apply as for the bioequivalence studies. The number of patients to be included in the study will depend on the variability of the target parameters and the acceptance range, and is usually much higher than the number of subjects in bioequivalence studies.

### 1.19.4 In-vitro Dissolution testing

Under certain circumstances, bioequivalence can be documented using in vitro approaches. For highly soluble, highly permeable, rapidly dissolving, orally administered drug products, documentation of bioequivalence using an in vitro approach (dissolution studies) is appropriate. In addition to the determination of the in-vivo performance, in vitro dissolution testing is an integral part of the assessment of bioequivalence, especially for the generic drug products. The comparative release profiles of the test and reference drug products are examined. The dissolution testing is conducted by a compendia method and the test product must pass the compendial specifications. For extended release products, the dissolution method and specifications are developed for each drug product. The specifications are applied only to that drug product to maintain its quality and manufacturing controls.

## 1.20. Objective of the Study

The use of metronidazole, 1-(2-hydroxyethyl)-2-methyl-5-nitroimidazole, has long been known for the treatment of trichomoniasis and more recently for the treatment of bacterial vaginosis. There are currently at least two effective ways to treat trichomoniasis or bacterial vaginosis with the administration of a metronidazole composition. In the first method, a single, large dose (~2 grams) of metronidazole is given as a bolus to the patient. The single treatment is clinically effective. A major drawback to the administration of single large dose metronidazole is the occurrence of significant and undesirable side effect such as nausea. A second and more generally accepted treatment entails orally administering 250 mgs of metronidazole three time a day for a period of 7 days. The lower dosage of metronidazole over a period of a week significantly reduces the occurrence and severity of side effect. However patient compliance is a problem can inadvertently forget to take one or more doses during the course of treatment, causing the plasma metronidazole level drop to bellow an acceptable therapeutic level for a period of several hours or more. The use of metronidazole is also known for the treatment of various other conditions, including amebiasis (acute amebic dysentry), and *Helicobecter*

77

*pylori* infection associated with duodenal disease. In order to reduce the number of daily doses of metronidazole needed to treat a microbial infection, while maintaining the benefit of making bioavailable effective amount of drug over an extended time period, it would be desirable to deliver a therapeutically effective amount of metronidazole in a once daily dose. Effectively maintaining acceptable bioavailability of metronidazole up to 24 hours with a single dose and without increased side effect relative to conventional multiple dose regimens cannot be accomplished simply by increasing the amount of active drug in a single dose. Metronidazole is aqueous soluble and is rapidly absorbed by the bloodstream. Metronidazole is also rapidly cleared from the bloodstream. Thus, merely administering increased amounts of immediate-release metronidazole results in a rapid peak, followed by a rapid decline in metronidazole levels. Such a profile is undesirable because of side effects caused by high peak levels of metronidazole. Also, the rapid clearing of the drug does not permit plasma metronidazole to remain at acceptable levels for 24 hours.

On the other hand, adding amounts of excipients in ratios typical of conventional modified release formulations which are presently available would result in a tablet which is too large for oral administration. For example, 750 mg of metronidazole represents at least about a 2-fold greater amount of active ingredient than is presently available in other pharmaceutical compositions which are available in modified release form. Moreover, metronidazole itself is not readily compressible, which presents a significant problem with respect to forming modified release tablets.

Thus, therefore objective of this study are-

> ➢ To provide an extended release metronidazole composition that will be capable of delivering acceptable bioavailability for up to 24 hours.

➢ To provide a composition this should be readily compressible such that the entire dose may be provided in a single tablet suitable for oral administration.

➢ Select such excepients (less than about 30% by weight) those must be capable of imparting both compressibility properties (for tabletting) and modified release properties (for bioavailability) in order to keep the size of a single tablet in the range of about 1000-1100 mg, while providing about 750 mg of metronidazole.

I hope that this study will capable of providing an extended release metronidazole composition that will be capable of delivering acceptable bioavailability for up to one day while maintaining all other properties of an ideal oral solid dosage form.

## 2. Materials and Methods

Using various proportions of Eudragit NM30D and Methocel Premium K4M, extended release formulations of Metronidazole were prepared separately through wet granulation. Eudragit NM30D and Methocel Premium K4M are dominant vehicles used for the preparation of oral controlled drug delivery systems. The matrix tablets were prepared by using ERWEKA TR-16 Compression machine (Germany) 16 station machine with 19.00 X 9.208 mm die, caplet, upper punches with embossed "M001" and lower punches with break line. Physical properties (hardness, thickness and friability) and release kinetics of those matrix tablets were studied. The dissolution was carried out in 'eight pocket ERWEKA tablet dissolution tester and twelve pockets Pharma test (USP Apparatus II) at pH 7.4. Comparisons are made of the effect of different excipients on the physical properties as well as zero order, First order, Higuchi, and Korsmeyer release kinetics of Metronidazole from Eudragit NM30D and Methocel Premium K4M.

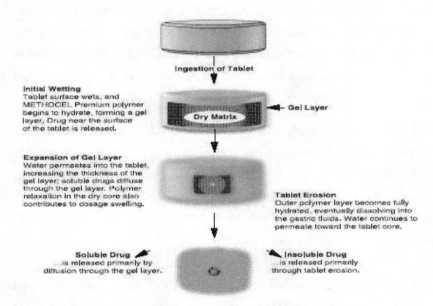

**Figure 2.1: Drug release from hydrophilic matrix tablet**

## 2.1 Materials used for Metronidazole Extended Release tablet

Metronidaoze was used as the active material for preparing mtronidazole extended release tablet. The active ingredient, rate -retarding polymer and other excipients are shown in the table 2.1.

**Table 2.1 List of polymers and other excipients used in preparation of matrix tablets**

| Name | Category | Source | Country of Origin |
|---|---|---|---|
| Metronidazole BP | Active | Alt Laboratory Limited | China |
| METHOCEL Premium K4M | Matrix forming agent | Colorcon Asia Pvt. Ltd | USA |
| Eudragit NM30D | Matrix forming agent | Evonik Rohm GmbH | Germany |
| Dimethicone | Antifoaming agent | Shenyang Jin Yi Lai Chemical Co. Ltd | China |
| Lactose Monohydrate BP | Filler | Foremost Farms | USA |
| Purified Talc BP | Lubricant | Merek | Germany |
| Colloidal Anhydrous Silica BP (Aerosil-200) | Glidant | Evonik Industries | Belgium |
| Magnesium stearate BP | Antiadherent | Peter Greven | Netherland |
| Opadry II 85G68918 | Coating Material | Colorcon Asia Pvt. Ltd | USA |
| FD & C Blue No-1 | Coloring agent | Sensient Color UK Ltd | USA |

## 2.1.1 Drug Profile

Metronidazole is an antimicrobial nitroimidazole derivative, which was originally introduced to treat Trichomonas vaginalis but nowadays is used for the treatment of anaerobic and protozoal infections. Metronidazole is bactericidal through toxic metabolites, which cause deoxyribonucleic acid (DNA) strand breakage. It has a bioavailability of more than 90% after oral administration. The drug is metabolized by the liver and the hydroxy-metabolite has also a therapeutic effect. Metronidazole was introduced in 1959 for the treatment of patients with Trichomonas vaginalis and it has since been evaluated in the treatment of infections caused by anaerobic bacteria. It is a member of the 5-nitroimidazole antimicrobials class, especially fatal on some protozoa. It has been used successfully in the treatment of vaginal infections, antibiotic- associated pseudomembranous colitis, trichomoniasis and symptomatic amebiasis. It is a drug of first choice in the infections of Helicobacter pylori5. It has also been reported to be of value in Crohn's disease. It is usually absorbed well (80-90%) by oral route. The principal route of elimination is hepatic oxidation and glucuronidation. Metronidazole has common adverse effects like nausea, diarrhea, anorexia, vomiting and urticaria, although it is widely used. The carcinogenic potential and effects on spermatogenesis are under investigation (Turgut *et al*, 2004).

## 2.1.1.1 Physicochemical Properties

Metronidazole is named as 2-methyl-5-nitroimidazole-1-ethanol or 1-(2 hydroxyethyl)-2-methyl-5-nitroimidazole. Its formula is $C_6H_9N_3O_3$ and the chemical formula can be seen in Figure. Molecular weight is 171.2 (BP, 2009).

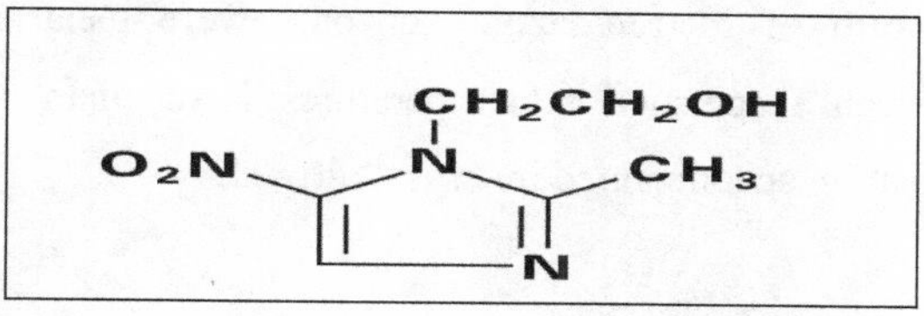

**Figure 2.2: Chemical Structure of Metronidazole**

It is white to pale yellow, odorless and in crystal or crystalline powder form, melting between 159-162°C. It is sparingly soluble in water, alcohol or chloroform and slightly soluble in ether. Its pKa was detected as 2.517 Metronidazole was reported to undergo hydrolysis in aqueous media due to the presence of photolytically generated hydroxyl radicals. Light irradiation has more effect on the degradation of metronidazole in solution than irradiation with sonic energy. Wang et al. studied the degradation kinetics under various conditions such as pH, total buffer concentration, ionic strength, temperature, light exposure and co-solvent system. The results indicated pseudofirst order degradation kinetics for metronidazole in aqueous solution. In the pH range between 3.9 and 3.6, metronidazole was more stable than in other pH regions. There was not enough degradation in a 50-day period for both light-exposed and light-protected samples. However, UV irradiation did accelerate the degradation processes of metronidazole in the light-exposed samples. The effect of gamma rays on metronidazole was investigated and it was found that gamma irradiation of metronidazole produced free radicals. In another study, metronidazole was found to become biologically inactive when it was impregnated into solid sensitivity discs and then exposed to light. The effect of light on parenteral solutions of metronidazole caused a fall in pH, an increase in nitrite ion concentration and formation of amber discoloration. From a thermodynamic study, it was concluded that aqueous suspensions of the anhydrous form of metronidazole benzoate were metastable and that storage of such suspension at temperatures lower than 38°C leads to hydrate formation accompanied by crystal growth

### 2.1.1.2 Pharmacology

Metronidazole and nitroimidazoles are thought to produce their bactericidal activity through four phases (Turgut *et al*, 2004).-

1. Entry into bacterial cell
2. Nitro group reduction
3. Action of the cytotoxic by products
4. Production of inactive end products

The selective toxicity of nitroimidazoles depends on two factors. The first is the reduction of nitroimidazoles. Since metronidazole is a small, lipophilic molecule that cannot ionize, it can easily enter into the microorganism cell with passive diffusion. Nitroimidazole sensitive cells are commonly anaerobic and include low redox potential proteins with a role in electron transfer. The second mechanism is to turn the nitro group of nitroimidazoles into intermediary toxic metabolites with the reduction caused by non-enzymatic chemical reactivity. This toxic metabolite interacts with DNA, RNA (ribonucleic acid) or intercellular proteins, but the major effect appears with the breakage of the DNA strand. Therefore, the inhibition of DNA synthesis causes the death of the cell. The therapeutic dose of the drug affects the lymphocytical DNA. Another mechanism is the self-reduction potential of nitroimidazoles that destroys intercellular electron transfer and depresses of NADH (nicotinamide adenine dinucleotide) and NADPH (nicotinamide adenine dinucleotide phosphate). As a result, the energy formation is inhibited. Both clinical and microbiological resistance has been demonstrated rarely. However, the study of Edwards et al. has shown that microorganisms like E. coli, Proteus and Klebsiella absorb metronidazole in the treatment of T. vaginalis. Therefore, the concentration of active substance in vaginal fluid has been decreased. The minimum effective concentration of metronidazole has been determined as 0.1-8 µg/ml, and general oral doses for 5 to 10 day treatment periods very between 400-800 mg. Serum concentration and dose range should be adjusted for newborns and children. The adjustment has been made according to body weight (35-50 mg/kg), because of the similarity of the clearance as in adults. There is no need to change the dose during pregnancy since there is not a significant difference in pharmacokinetics. The drug can be administrated by intravenous infusion with a rate of 5 mL/min. every 8 hours (h), if the oral route is not available. Metronidazole can be administered rectally 1 g, 3 times a day for 3 days. The oral dose in acute ulcerative gingivitis is 600 mg per day. The drug can be given at a dose of 500 mg for 7 days vaginally. Solutions of 1% and gels at different ratios have also been used. It has been reported that 500mg metronidazole can be effective topically, once or twice a day (Welling *et al.*,1972).

### 2.1.1.3 Pharmacokinetics

**Absorption**

The oral absorption of metronidazole is excellent, with bioavailability often reported as >90%. The peak plasma drug concentration ($C_{max}$) after a single dose of 500mg is approximately 8 to 13 mg/L, with a corresponding time ($t_{max}$) of 0.25 to 4 hours.

**Distribution**

Metronidazole has generally been reported to have good penetration into the cerebrospinal fluid (CSF) and central nervous system (CNS). A patient with Fusobacterium meningitis had CSF concentrations of 13.9 and 11 mg/L at 2 and 8 hour, respectively, after oral administration of 500 mg doses twice daily. Protein binding of metronidazole is less than 20%. The reported volumes of distribution ($V_d$) in various studies have ranged from 0.65 to 0.71 L/kg in newborn infants, to 0.51 to 1.1 L/kg in adults. Single dose studies with oral and intravenous 500 mg metronidazole have determined the area under the serum concentration-time curve (AUC) to be approximately 100-159 mg/L. Pregnant women tend to have AUCs that also fall in this range, but children and infants may have higher AUCs depending on the dose utilized.

**Metabolism**

Metronidazole is metabolized in the liver into two major metabolites. These are (1-(2-hydroxy-ethy)-2-hydroxy-methyl-5-nitroimidazole)) hydroxy-metronidazole and 2-methyl-2-nitroimidazole-1-acetic acid. The acetic acid metabolite is only found in urine and does not possess any pharmacological activity. However, hydroxy-metronidazole has an antimicrobial potency approximately 30% that of metronidazole against certain strains of bacteria and can be detected readily in the systemic circulation. The acetic acid metabolite has only 5% of the activity of the

86

parent drug and is only detectable in patients with renal dysfunction. Glucuronide and sulfate conjugates and an oxidation product have also been detected. The metabolization tract and chemical formulas can be seen in Figure 2.3.

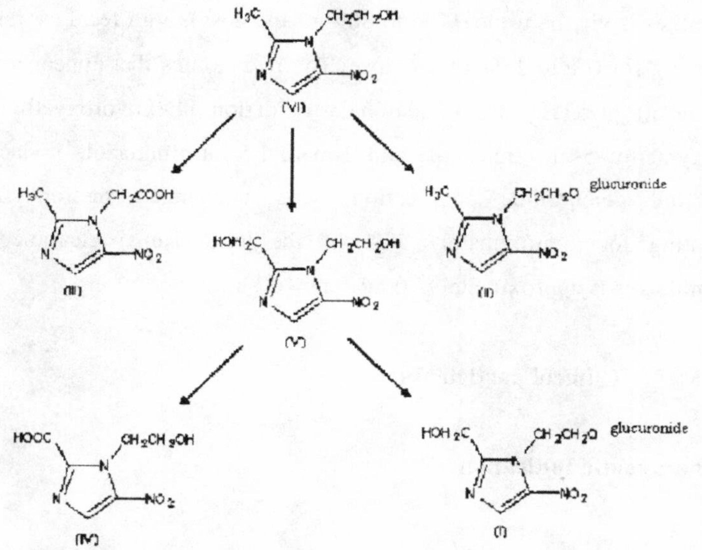

Figure 2.3: The metabolism pathway of metronidazole in humans and chemical structure of metabolites (Turgut *et al*, 2004).

VI: Metronidazole

V: 1-(2-hydroxyethyl)-2-hydroxymethyl-5-nitro-imidazole;

IV: 1-(2-hydroxyethyl)-2-carboxylic acid-5 nitro-imidazole;

III: 1-acetic acid-2-methyl-5-nitroimidazole;

I and II are glucuronide conjugates.

87

**Elimination**

Disposition of metronidazole in the body is similar for both oral and intravenous dosage forms, with an average elimination half-life in healthy humans of 8 hours. The major route of elimination of metronidazole and its metabolites is via the urine (60% to 80% of the dose), with fecal excretion accounting for 6% to 15% of the dose. The metabolites that appear in the urine result primarily from side-chain oxidation [1-(ßhydroxyethyl)-2-hydroxymethyl-5-nitroimidazole and 2-methyl-5-nitroimidazole-1-ylacetic acid] and glucuronide conjugation, with unchanged metronidazole accounting for approximately 20% of the total. Renal clearance of metronidazole is approximately 10 mL/ min/1.73m$^2$.

### 2.1.1.5    Clinical particulars

#### a) Therapeutic Indication

Metronidazole is indicated for the treatment of:

**Bacterial**

- Bacterial vaginosis, commonly associated with overgrowth of *Gardnerella,* species and coinfective anaerobes (Mobiluncus, Bacteroides), in symptomatic patients.
- Pelvic inflammatory disease in conjunction with other antibiotics such as ofloxacin, levofloxacin, or ceftriaxone.
- Anaerobic infections such as *Bacteroides fragilis, spp, Fusobacterium spp, Clostridium spp, Peptostreptococcus spp, Prevotella spp*, or any other anaerobes in intra-abdominal abscess,

peritonitis, diverticulitis, empyema, pneumonia, aspiration pneumonia, lung abscess, diabetic foot ulcer, meningitis and brain abscesses, bone and joint infections, septicemia, endometritis, or endocarditis.

- Pseudomembranous colitis due to *Clostridium difficile.*
- *Helicobacter pylori* eradication therapy, as part of a multi-drug regimen in peptic ulcer disease (Sutter *et al.,* 1979)

## Protozoal

**Amoebiasis:** Infections caused by *Entamoeba histolytica.*

**Giardiasis:** Infection of the small intestine caused by the ingestion of infective cysts of protozoan *Giardia lamblia.* Trichomoniasis: infection caused by *Trichomonas vaginalis*, which is a common cause of vaginitis and is the most frequently presenting new infection of the common sexually transmitted diseases.

## Nonspecific

- Prophylaxis for those undergoing potentially contaminated colorectal surgery or appendectomies and may be combined with neomycin
- Acute gingivitis and other dental infections (TGA approved, non-U.S. Food and Drug Administration (FDA) approved)
- Crohn's disease with colonic or perianal involvement (non-FDA approved) – believed to be more effective in combination with ciprofloxacin
- Topical metronidazole is indicated for the treatment of rosacea, and in the treatment of malodorous fungating wounds.

- Also used in cases of malodorous and almost-constant flatulence (Simms-Cendan, 1996).

**Preterm births**

Metronidazole has also been used in women to prevent preterm birth associated with bacterial vaginosis, amongst other risk factors including the presence of cervicovaginal fetal fibronectin (fFN). A randomised controlled trial demonstrated that metronidazole was ineffective in preventing preterm delivery in high-risk pregnant women and, conversely, the incidence of preterm delivery was actually higher in women treated with metronidazole. Lamont has argued that Metronidazole is not the right antibiotic to administer in these circumstances and was often administered too late to be of use. Clindamycin administered early in the second trimester to women who test positive for bacterial vaginosis seems to be more effective (Shennan *et al.*, 2006)

**b) Contraindications**

Metronidazole is contraindicated in patients with a prior history of hypersensitivity to Metronidazole or other nitroimidazole derivatives. In patients with trichomoniasis, Metronidazole is contraindicated during the first trimester of pregnancy.

**c) Adverse Reactions**

The most serious adverse reactions reported in patients treated with Metronidazole have been convulsive seizures, encephalopathy, aseptic meningitis, optic and peripheral neuropathy, the latter characterized mainly by numbness or paresthesia of an extremity. Since persistent peripheral neuropathy has been reported in some patients receiving prolonged administration of Metronidazole, patients should be specifically warned about these reactions and should be told to stop the drug and report immediately to their physicians if any neurologic symptoms occur.

The most common adverse reactions reported have been referable to the gastrointestinal tract, particularly nausea reported by about 12% of patients, sometimes accompanied by headache, anorexia, and occasionally vomiting; diarrhea; epigastric distress; and abdominal cramping. Constipation has also been reported.

The following reactions have also been reported during treatment with Metronidazole:

**Mouth:** A sharp, unpleasant metallic taste is not unusual. Furry tongue, glossitis, and stomatitis have occurred; these may be associated with a sudden overgrowth of Candida which may occur during therapy.

**Hematopoietic**: Reversible neutropenia (leukopenia); rarely, reversible thrombocytopenia.

**Cardiovascular:** Flattening of the T-wave may be seen in electrocardiographic tracings.

**Central Nervous System:** Encephalopathy, aseptic meningitis, convulsive seizures, optic neuropathy, peripheral neuropathy, dizziness, vertigo, incoordination, ataxia, confusion, dysarthria, irritability, depression, weakness, and insomnia.

**Hypersensitivity:** Urticaria, erythematous rash, Stevens-Johnson Syndrome, toxic epidermal necrolysis, flushing, nasal congestion, dryness of the mouth (or vagina or vulva), and fever.

**Renal:** Dysuria, cystitis, polyuria, incontinence, and a sense of pelvic pressure. Instances of darkened urine have been reported by approximately one patient in 100,000. Although the pigment which is probably responsible for this phenomenon has not been positively identified, it is almost certainly a metabolite of Metronidazole and seems to have no clinical significance.

**Other:** Proliferation of Candida in the vagina, dyspareunia, decrease of libido, proctitis, and fleeting joint pains sometimes resembles "serum sickness." If patients receiving Metronidazole drink alcoholic beverages, they may experience abdominal distress, nausea, vomiting, flushing, or headache. A modification of the taste of alcoholic beverages has also been reported. Rare cases of pancreatitis, which generally abated on withdrawal of the drug, have been reported.

Crohn's disease patients are known to have an increased incidence of gastrointestinal and certain extraintestinal cancers. There have been some reports in the medical literature of breast and colon cancer in Crohn's disease patients who have been treated with Metronidazole at high doses for extended periods of time. A cause and effect relationship has not been established. Crohn's disease is not an approved indication for Metronidazole.

### 2.1.2 Excepient Profile

### A) Eudragit NM30D

Eudragit NM 30 D is the aqueous dispersion of a neutral copolymer based on ethyl acrylate and methyl methacrylate (www.evonik.com).

*Physical properties:* It is a milky-white liquid of low viscosity with a faint characteristic odors.

*Product Form:* Aqueous Dispersion 30%

*Chemical structure:*

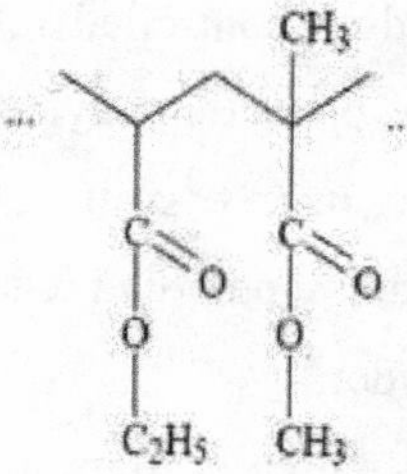

**Figure 2.4: Chemical Structure of Eudragit NM30D**

*Targeted Drug Release Area:* Time controlled release, pH independent

*Dissolution:*

- Insoluble
- Low permeability
- pH independent swelling

*Characteristics:*

- No plasticizer required
- Highly flexible
- Suitable for matrix structure

**B) Methocel Premium K4M**

METHOCEL (Trademark of the Dow Chemical Company) cellulose ethers are water-soluble polymers derived from cellulose, the most abundant polymer in nature. These products have been used as key ingredients in pharmaceutical and other applications for over 50 years (www.colorcon.com). Of all drug forms, patients overwhelmingly prefer solid oral dosage and hydrophilic matrix systems are among the most widely used means of providing controlled release in solid oral dosage form. METHOCEL (Hydroxypropyl methylcellulose) as the controlled release agent in hydrophilic matrix systems offers a wide range of properties, consistent high quality and broad regulatory approval.

***Physical form***: off-white powder.

***Particle size***: Premium grades – 99% < 40 mesh screen

**Table 2.2: Description of Methocel Premium K4M**

| Methocel Premium Product Grade | Specification | Methocel Premium K4M |
|---|---|---|
| Methoxyl,% | USP | 19-24 |
| Hydroxypropoxyl,% | USP | 7-12 |
| Substitution type | USP/EP | 2208 |
| Chlorides,max, % | EP | 0.5 |
| Apparent viscosity, 2% In water at $20^0$C, cP | USP | 3000-5600 |
| Apparent viscosity, 2% In water at $20^0$C, mPa s | EP | 2308-3755 |
| pH, 1% in water | EP | 5.5-8.0 |
| Loss on drying, max % | USP/ EP | 5.0 |

| Organic impurities, volatile | USP | Pass |
|---|---|---|
| Residue in ignition, max,% | USP | 1.5 |
| Ash, sulfated, max% | EP | 1.0 |
| Heavy metals, as Pb, max, ppm | USP/ EP | 10 |
| Solution color, yellowness, 1% in water | EP | Pass |

## C) Dimethicone

Dimethicone (also called polymethylsiloxane) is a silicon-based polymer used as a lubricant and conditioning agent.

*Function/use(s):* Antifoaming Agent, Skin-Conditioning Agent – Occlusive, Skin Protectant, Emollient, Skin conditioning, Skin protecting.

## D) Lactose Monohydrate BP

Lactose Monohydrate is a natural disaccharide, obtained from milk, which consists of one glucose and one galactose moiety. Lactose Monohydrate may be modified as to its physical characteristics. It may contain varying proportions of amorphous lactose. Lactose occurs as white to off-white crystalline particles or powder. Several different brands of anhydrous lactose are commercially available which contain anhydrous β-lactose and anhydrous α-lactose. Anhydrous lactose typically contains 70–80% anhydrous b-lactose and 20–30% anhydrous α-lactose.

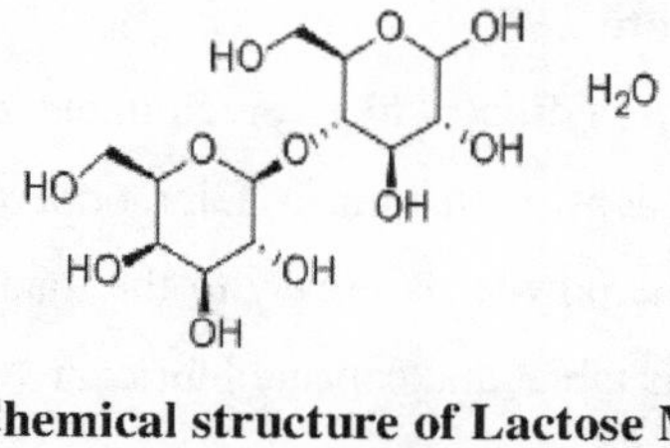

**Figure 2.5: Chemical structure of Lactose Monohydrate**

Lactose monohydrate used as binding agent; directly compressible tableting excipient, lyophilization aid, tablet and capsule filler (Rowe *et al.,* 2006).

### E) Purified Talc

Talc is very fine hydrous magnesium calcium silicate, white to grayish-white, odorless, impalpable, unctuous, crystalline powder. It adheres readily to the skin and is soft to the touch and free from grittiness. It is used as anticaking agent; glidant; tablet and capsule diluent; tablet and capsule lubricant.

### F) Colloidal silicon dioxide (Aerosil 200)

Colloidal silicon dioxide is submicroscopic fumed silica with a particle size of about 15 nm. It is a light, loose, bluish-white colored, odorless, tasteless, nongritty amorphous powder (Rowe *et al.,* 2006). It is widely used in pharmaceuticals. Its small particle size and large specific surface area give it desirable flow characteristics which are exploited to improve the flow properties of dry powders in a number of processes, e.g, tableting (www.colorcon.com).

### G) Magnesium Stearate

Magnesium Stearate is a fine, white, precipitated or milled, impalpable powder or low bulk density, having a faint odor of stearic acid and a characteristic taste. The powder is greasy to the touch and readily adheres to the skin. It is used as tablet and capsule lubricant.

## 2.2 Equipments

List of equipments used in the preparation and characterization of extended release Metronidazole tablets are given in the Table 2.3.

**Table 2.3: List of Equipments used in the preparation and characterization of matrix tablets**

| Name | Manufacturer | Country of origin |
|---|---|---|
| Electric balance | Sartorius, CPA225D | Germany |
| | Sartorius AG | Germany |
| | OHAUS LS 200 | Switzerland |
| Sieve | Endecotts test sieve | UK |
| Compression machine | ERWEKA TR-16 | Germany |
| Electronic Hardness tester | Sotax HT10 | Switzerland |
| Halogen moisture analyzer | OHAUS-MB45 | Switzerland |
| Friability tester | Electrolab, EF-1W | India |
| Digital Bulk density apparatus | Sunita Impex Private Ltd | India |
| Fluid bed dryer | Laboratory FBD FB-15 | Thiland |
| Tray dryer | Memment | Germany |
| Coating Machine | Pam Glatt | India |

## 2.3 Preparation of Metronidazole Extended Release Tablet

## 2.3.1 Preparation of extended release Metronidazole tablet using Eudragit NM30D as matrix forming agent:

Formula U-1, U-2 and U-3 were proposed for preparation of Metronidazole Extended release formulation using Eudragit as release retardant and matrix forming agent.

### *Dispensing*

Here the items are dispensed as per Table 3.3 for a batch size 2000 tablets. During dispensing active (Metronidazole BP) was dispensed considering potency of the active and the batch weight remains constant by compensating with Lactose Monohydrate. For this purpose active and Lactose Monohydrate BP are calculated as per bellowing equation:

(1)    Calculate Quantity of Metronidazole BP as follows:

$$\text{Quantity of Metronidazole BP} = \frac{\text{Theoretical Quantity x 100}}{\text{Potency of Metronidazole BP}}$$

(2)    Calculated quantity of Lactose  Monohydrate BP as follows :

Quantity of Lactose Monohydrate BP = ( Quantity of Metronidazole and Lactose Monohydrate BP – X)gm

Every item except Eudragit NM30D is dispensed in food grade poly bags and tight with rubber tie. Eudragit NM30D is dispensed in beaker and the beaker is kept rapped with food grade poly bag tight with rubber.

**Table 2.4: Formulation for Metronidazole extended release tablet having Eudragit NM30D matrices**

| Name of Materials | Quantity Per Tablet (mg/Tablet) | | |
|---|---|---|---|
| | U-1 | U-2 | U-3 |
| Metronidazole BP | 600 | 600 | 600 |
| Lactose monohydrate BP | 61.65 | 58.65 | 55.65 |
| Eudragit NM30D | 0.03ml (9mg) | 0.04ml (12mg) | 0.05ml (15mg) |
| Dimethicone | 0.3 | 0.3 | 0.3 |
| Purified Talc | 6 | 6 | 6 |
| Metronidazole BP | 150 | 150 | 150 |
| Lactose monohydrate BP | 170 | 170 | 170 |
| Magnesium Stearate BP | 2.05 | 2.05 | 2.05 |
| Colloidal Anhydrous silica BP | 1 | 1 | 1 |

*NB: Eudragit NM30D contain 30% solid as w/v.*

*Granulation*

First portion of the Lactose Monohydrate BP and Metronidazole BP were loaded in a poly bag and then passed through a 500 micron sieve. Granules were dry mixed for one minute. Purified Talc after sieving through 500 micron screen was added with Eudragit NM30D and Dimethicone in a beaker. Purified water was added in the beaker and stirrer for about 15 minutes to prepare slurry. This slurry was then mixed with already mixed Metronidazole BP and Lactose Monohydrate BP. These materials were mixed until getting satisfactory mass. Then the materials were loaded into tray dryer and dried at 70°C to get moisture content bellow 2-3%. 4/5 portion (1083.12 gm) of the granules were passed 25 mesh (710 micron) screen and rest of the material (270.78 gm) were passed through 18 mesh (1 mm) screen and loaded into a poly bag. Second portion of the Lactose Moohydrate BP and Metronidazole BP and Colloidal Anhydrous Silica (Aerosil-200) were sieved through 500 micron screen, added in the poly bag and blended for 1 minute. Finally Magnesium Stearate BP was added with the granules and again blended for 1 minute.

*Compression*

Previously prepared granules were compressed for desired tablet with specific weight, shape and hardness. For this purpose ERWEKA compression machine was set with 19 X 9.208 mm caplet shaped punch and die set. Upper punches have embossed "M001" and lower punch have break line. Compression was controlled such to keep the target weight 1000mg ± 3% , thickness range 6.40 mm to 6.80 mm and hardness above 10 Kp.

**Table 2.5: Tablet Tooling Description**

| Parameter | Value |
|---|---|
| Shape | Caplet |
| Size | 19.00 X 9.208 mm |
| Upper Punches | Embossed " M001" |
| Lower Punches | Break Line |

**Table 2.6: Machine Control**

| Stage | Parameter | Value |
|---|---|---|
| Pre Compression | Insertion Depth | 1.32 mm |
| | Edge Thickness | 2.50 mm |
| Main Compression | Insertion Depth | 3.00 mm |
| Main Compression | Edge Thickness | 3.50 mm |
| | Fill Camm | 14 mm |
| | Feeder Speed | 15 RPM |
| | Dosing | 7.5 mm |
| General | Production Speed | 25 RPM |
| | Tabs Per Hour | 400TPM |
| | Effective Punches | 16 Nos |

**Table 2.7: Compression Force Limits**

| Parameter | Value |
|---|---|
| S+ ( Single Punch Max. Value ) | 22 KN |
| M+ ( Max. Mean Value ) | 20.5 KN |
| M set ( Mean Value ) | 16.3 KN |
| M- ( Min. Mean Value ) | 12 KN |
| S- ( Single Punch Min. Value ) | 10.0 KN |
| Srel | .03 % |
| Max Punch Load | 22 KN |

*Coating:*

Tablets are film coated with a color solution using Opadry II 85G68918 and FD & C Blue No-1. All the preparations were stored in airtight containers at room temperature for further study

## 2.3.2 Preparation of extended release Metronidazole Tablet using Methocel Premium K4M as matrix forming agent:

Formula M-1, M-2, M-3, M-4 and M-5 were proposed for preparation of Metronidazole Extended release formulation using Methocel Premium K4M as release retardant and matrix forming agent.

### Dispensing

Here the items are dispensed as per Table 3.4 for a batch size 2000 tablets. During dispensing active (Metronidazole BP) was dispensed considering potency of the active and the batch weight remains constant by compensating with Lactose Monohydrate.

**Table 2.8: Formulation for Metronidazole extended release tablet having Methocel Premium K4M matrices**

| Name of Materials | Quantity Per Tablet (mg/Tablet) | | | | |
|---|---|---|---|---|---|
| | M-1 | M-2 | M-3 | M-4 | M-5 |
| Metronidazole BP | 750 | 750 | 750 | 750 | 750 |
| Lactose monohydrate BP | 314.85 | 309.85 | 306.35 | 304.85 | 299.85 |
| Methocel Premium K4M | 30 | 35 | 38.5 | 40 | 45 |
| Colloidal Anhydrous silica BP | 2.75 | 2.75 | 2.75 | 2.75 | 2.75 |
| Magnesium Stearate BP | 2.4 | 2.4 | 2.4 | 2.4 | 2.4 |

## Granulation:

Lactose Monohydrate BP Metronidazole BP were taken in a poly bag and then passed through a 500 micron sieve and loaded in RMG. Granules were dry mixed for one minute. Purified water was added and mixed until getting satisfactory mass. Then the materials were loaded into FBD and dried at 70°C to get moisture content bellow 1.5-2%. 1/3 portion (approx. 730 gm) of the granules were passed 12 mesh (1.7 mm) screen and rest of the material (approx. 1460 gm) were passed through 18 (1 mm) mesh screen and loaded into a poly bag. Colloidal Anhydrous Silica (Aerosil-200) was sieved through 500 micron screen, added in the poly bag and blended for 1 minute. Finally Magnesium Stearate BP was added with the granules and again blended for 1 minute.

## Compression

Previously prepared granules were compressed for desired tablet with specific weight, shape and hardness. For this purpose ERWEKA compression machine was set with 19 X 9.208 mm caplet shaped punch and die set. Upper punches have embossed "M001" and lower punch have break line. Compression was controlled such to keep the target weight 1100 mg ± 3% , thickness range 6.75 mm to 7.00 mm and hardness above 10 Kp

**Table 2.9: Tooling Description**

| Parameter | Value |
|---|---|
| Shape | Caplet |
| Size | 19.00 X 9.208 mm |
| Upper Punches | Embossed " M001" |
| Lower Punches | Break Line |

**Table 2.10: Machine Control**

| Stage | Parameter | Value |
|---|---|---|
| Pre Compression | Insertion Depth | 1.32 mm |
| | Edge Thickness | 2.50 mm |
| Main Compression | Insertion Depth | 3.00 mm |
| Main Compression | Edge Thickness | 3.50 mm |
| | Fill Camm | 14 mm |
| | Feeder Speed | 15 RPM |
| | Dosing | 8.3 mm |
| General | Production Speed | 25 RPM |
| | Tabs Per Minute | 400TPM |
| | Effective Punches | 16 Nos |

**Table 2.11: Compression Force Limits**

| Parameter | Value |
|---|---|
| S+ ( Single Punch Max. Value ) | 22 KN |
| M+ ( Max. Mean Value ) | 20.4 KN |
| M set ( Mean Value ) | 18.5 KN |
| M- ( Min. Mean Value ) | 16 KN |
| S- ( Single Punch Min. Value ) | 10.5 KN |
| Srel | .05 % |
| Max Punch Load | 22 KN |

*Coating*

104

Tablets are film coated with a color solution using Opadry II 85G68918 and FD & C Blue No-1. All the preparations were stored in airtight containers at room temperature for further study.

## 2.4 Evaluation of Powders

The powders were evaluated for angle of repose, loose bulk density, tapped bulk density, compressibility index, and total porosity (Mourya *et al.,*2010).

### 2.4.1 Moisture Content

Moisture content of the granule was determined using Halogen moisture analyzer. For that purpose One gram (1g) of the granules was put into the drying chamber of the moisture analyzer and dried at constant temperature until constant weight is observed. The moisture content (MC) was deduced as difference between the initial ($W_o$) and final weight ($W_f$) of the granules, expressed as a percentage and calculated as:

$$MC= \{(W_o-W_f) / W_o\} \times 100$$

### 2.4.2 Bulk Density

LBD ( Loose Bulk Density ) and TBD (Tapped Bulk Density) were determined by 5 g of powder from each formula, previously lightly shaken to break agglomerates formed, was placed into a 50 ml measuring cylinder. After that initial volume was observed, the cylinder was allowed to fall under its own weight onto a hard surface from the height of 2 cm at 2 second intervals. The reading of tapping was continued until no further change in volume was noted. Using the following equation LBD and TBD was calculated:

LBD = weight of the powder / volume of the packing.

TBD = weight of the powder / Tapped volume of the packing.

### 2.4.3 Compressibility Index

A quantity of 5 g of powder from each formula, previously lightly shaken to break any agglomerates formed, was introduced into a Pharmatest Densitometer (Germany) with 50 ml measuring cylinder. After the initial volume was observed, the cylinder was allowed to fall under its own weight onto a hard surface from the height of 2 cm at 2 seconds intervals. The tapping was continued until no further change in volume was noted. The compressibility index of the granules was determined by Carr's compressibility index:

Carr' Index ( % ) = { ( TBD – LBD ) x 100 } / TBD

### 2.4.4 Angle of Repose

The angle of repose of granules was determined by the funnel method. The accurately weighed granules were taken in a funnel. The height of the funnel was adjusted in such a way that the tip of the funnel just touched the apex of the heap of the granules. The granules were allowed to flow through the funnel freely onto the surface. The diameter of the powder cone was measured and the angle of repose was calculated using the following equation:

Angle of Repose $\theta = \tan^{-1} h/r$

Where, h = Height of the powder cone.

"r" = Radius of the powder cone

### 2.5 Evaluation of Tablets

### 2.5.1 Hardness

Five tablets of each of the formulations were taken and hardness was measured by Hardness tester (Sotax HT10, Switzerland). The average value was calculated and the testing unit was Kilopond (Kp).

## 2.5.2 Thickness

Six tablets of each of the formulations were taken and thickness was measured by Thickness tester (Sotax HT10, Switzerland). The values were reported in millimeter (mm).

## 2.5.3 Friability

Ten tablets of each of the formulations were weighed out and taken into the rotating disk of a Friability Tester (Pharmatest, Germany). It was allowed to rotate at 25 rpm for 4 minutes (100 revolutions). At the end of the rotation, tablets were collected, dedusted and reweighed. The friability was calculated as the percent of weight loss.

$$\text{Friability} = \frac{\text{Weight Loss}}{\text{Initial Weight}} \times 100$$

## 2.5.4 Drug Content Assay

20 tablets were weighed and powdered. A quantity of powder containing 0.2 gm of metronidazole was transferred to a sintered glass crucible and extract with six 10 ml quantities of hot acetone. Cool, add to the combined extracts 50 ml of acetic anhydride and 0.1 ml of a 1% w/v solution of brilliant green in anhydrous acetic acid and titrate with 0.1 M perchloric acid VS to a yellowish-green end point. Operation was repeated without powdered tablets. The difference between the titrations represents the

amount of perchloric acid required. Each ml of 0.1 m perchloric acid VS is equivalent to 17.12 mg of Metronidazole.

$$\text{Calculation:} \quad \frac{\text{Titrate volume X Factor X Eq. Wt. X Average W}}{\text{Sample wt in mg}} \ \text{mg}$$

## 2.6 In-Vitro Dissolution Study of Metronidazole Extended Release Tablets

### *Dissolution Test*

Dissolution Set Up: "The Rotating Paddle Method" consists of a paddle held by a motor shaft. The sinker is used to hold the sample immersed into the dissolution medium. The entire flask is immersed in a constant – temperature bath set at 37°c. The temperature range is maintained at 37°C ± 0.5°C. The rotating speed and the position of the basket must meet specific requirements set forth in the current USP.

### *Dissolution Medium*

All dissolution studies were carried out for extended release Metronidazole formulations according to USP II. 0.1N HCl was used as dissolution medium. The amount of drug dissolved in the medium was determined by UV spectrophotometer at 278 nm.

### *Standard Solution preparation*

44.50 mg Metronidazole WS was weighed accurately in a volumetric flask.50-60 ml 0.1N Hydrochloric acid was added and sonicated it in ultrasonic bath for 10 minutes to dissolve and make volume with the same and mix. 2 ml of this solution was diluted to 50 ml with the 0.1N Hydrochloric acid and mixed.

### Sample Solution preparation

900 ml dissolution medium was taken into 6 vessels each and maintained temperature $37\pm0.5°C$. One tablet each was placed in 6 individual vessels. To exclude air bubbles from the surface of the tablet care was taken, immediately operate the apparatus at 100 rpm. 5 ml from each vessel was pipetted at $1^{st}$ $2^{nd}$, $4^{th}$, $6^{th}$, $8^{th}$ $10^{th}$ and $12^{th}$ hours from starting time and each time solution were replaced with fresh medium.

### 2.7 Data Treatment

To analyze the *in vitro* release data various model dependent kinetic models i.e. Zero Order Plotting, First Order Plotting, Higutchi and Korsmeyer-Peppas Plotting were used to describe the release kinetics and model independent method i.e, similarity factor $f_2$ and difference factor $f_1$ were used to compare the release profile of proposed formulations with the patent drug Flagyl ER Tablet.

### 2.7.1 Mathematical expression of drug release mechanism from controlled release dosage from

The release of drug from controlled dosage form is controlled by several processes. These are extraction or diffusion of drug from matrix and erosion of matrix alternatively; drug may be dissolved in the matrix material and be released by diffusion through membrane. Matrices may be prepared from soluble, insoluble or erodable materials. In some cases drug may be released by osmotic process.

### Diffusion

The release of drug is determined by the diffusion through the polymeric membrane. It can be mathematically expressed as –

$$J = -D \, dc/dx \dots\dots\dots\dots\dots (1)$$

Here,

J    = Flux of drug in amount/area – time

D    = Diffusion coefficient in area/time

C    = Concentration

X    = Diffusion path length

Assuming Steady-state level, equation (1) can be integrated as

$$J = - D \, C/I$$

When water insoluble membrane is employed then the equation is

$$dM/dt = - ADK\Delta C/I$$

Where,

dM/dt       = the amount of drug that diffuses

A = cross sectional area

K = partition coefficient

I  = diffusion path length

$\Delta C$   = the concentration gradient across the membrane

### First order release mechanism

Most sustained release formulation tends to give first order release pattern. This release equation is based on Fick's law, described as

$$dc/dt = - DA. \, (C_m - C_r)/h$$

Where

dc/dt = the mass of drug which diffuses in unit time

A = cross sectional area

D = diffusion constant

$C_m$ = the initial concentration in the dosage form

$C_r$ = the concentration in the dissolution me

H = thickness of the barrier

Under sink condition, the equation becomes

$$dC_m/dt = - K_t C_m$$

Where,

$K_t$ = constant

Integration of the above equation gives the first order equation

$$Log\ C_m = log\ C^o_m - kt/2.303$$

Where,

$C_m$ = the concentration at time t

K = the first order release rate constant

## Zero order release mechanism

A zero order release of drug is needed for the dosage form, which means that the rate of drug is independent of drug concentration, expressed by the following equations.

$$dc/dt = k_{ro}$$

or

$$dM/dt = k_{ro}$$

At times it is not possible to generate a constant release product and a slow first-order release of drug is employed.

## Higuchi release mechanism

111

Obviously, for this system to be diffusion controlled the rate of dissolution of drug particles within the matrix must be much faster than the diffusion rate of dissolute drug leaving the matrix. Deviation of mathematical model to describe this system involves the following assumption (Higuchi, 1963).

a) A pseudo-steady state is maintained during drug release

b) The diameter of drug particles is less than the average distance of drug dissolution through the matrix

c) The bathing solution provides sink conditions at all times

d) The diffusion coefficient of drug in the matrix remains constant, (i.e. no change occurs in the characteristics of the polymer matrix)

Higuchi has derived the rate of release of drugs dispersed in an inert matrix system.

This equation is -

$$dM/dh = C_o.dh - C_s/2$$

Where,

dM = Change in the amount of drug release per unit area

dh = Change in the thickness of the zone of matrix that been depleted of the          drug

$C_o$ = Total amount of drug in a unit volume of the matrix

$C_s$ = Sustained concentration of the drug within the matrix

### *Bioequivalence Analysis*

*In vitro* release profile of the reference Metronidazole BP extended release (ER) tablets, (Flagyl ER, Pfizer) was performed under similar conditions as used for *in vitro* release testing of the test product for the release of Metronidazole (Laila *et al.*, 2009). The difference factors similarity factors between the formulations were determined using the data obtained from the drug release studies. The data were analyzed by the formula shown in Equation.

$$f_1 = \frac{\sum [R_t - T_t]}{\sum R_t} \times 100$$

$$f_2 = 50 \log \{[1 + (1/N) \sum (R_t - T_t)]^{-0.5} \times 100\}$$

Where,

N = Number of time points,

$R_t$ and $T_t$ = Dissolution of reference and test products at time t respectively.

$f_1$ = Difference factor.

$f_2$ = Similarity factor.

If $f_1$ is less than 15 and $f_2$ is greater than 50 it is considered that 2 products share similar drug release behaviors.

## 2.7.2 Plots used to explain data

Cumulative % drug release vs. time ( Zero-order Kinetic Model); Log cumulative of % remaining vs time ( First order kinetic model); cumulative % drug release vs. square root of time ( Higuchi model ) and Log cumulative of % remaining vs log of time (Korsmeyer-Peppas Plotting).

## 2.7.3 Mechanism of Drug Release

Korsmeyer *et a.,l* ( 1983 ) derived a simple relationship which described drug release from a polymeric system. To find out the mechanism of drug release, first 60% drug release data was fitted in Korsmeyer-Peppas model:

$Mt / M\alpha = Ktn$ ..................... (4)

Where, $M_t / M_\alpha$ is the fraction of drug released at time t, k is the rate constant and n is the release exponent. The n value is used to characterize different release mechanism as given in the following table for cylindrical shaped matrices:

**Table 2.12: Diffusion exponent and solute release mechanism for cylindrical shape**

| Diffusion exponent (n) | Overall solute diffusion mechanism |
|---|---|
| 0.45 | Fickian diffusion |
| 0.45 < n < 0.89 | Anomalous (non-Fickian) diffusion |
| 0.89 | Case – II transport. |
| n> 0.89 | Super case-II transport. |

## 3. Results and Discussion

The present study was designed to develop extended release tablets of Metronidazole by using Eudragit NM30D and Methocel Premium K4M as rate retarding factor separately by wet granulation method. Eudragit NM30D was used in the proposed formulations U-1 to U-3 and Methocel Premium K4M in M-1 to M-5 in order to evaluate the amount of polymer required to provide desired release rate for 24 hours period. The powders of proposed formulations were evaluated for Moisture content, LBD, TBD, Compressibility index, Angle of repose and drug content (Table: 3.1).

### 3.1 Evaluation of Granules

### 3.1.1 Moisture Content

Moisture content of the granules for formulation U-1 to U-3 ranged from 2.32 to 2.87 and for formulation M-1 to M-5 ranged from 1.63 to 1.85

### 3.1.2 Loose and Tapped Bulk Density

The results of LBD and TBD ranged from $0.45 \pm 0.04$ to $0.51 \pm 0.04$ and $0.55 \pm 0.03$ to $0.62 \pm 0.01$ respectively.

### 3.1.3 Compressibility index (%)

The results of compressibility index (%) ranged from $14.55 \pm 0.02$ to $20.34 \pm 0.04$.

### 3.1.4 Angles of repose

The results of angles of repose ranged from 19.64±0.02 to 23.15 ± 0.03 (°).

### 3.1.5 Drug content

The drug content in a weighed amount of all formulations ranged from 98.94% to 100.21%. All these results indicate that the granules possess satisfactory flow properties, compressibility and drug content.

**Table 3.1 Properties of granules of Metronidazole containing Eudragit NM30D and Methocel Premium K4M as release retardant.**

| Formulations | Loose Bulk Density (LBD) (g/ml) | Tapped Bulk Density (TBD) (g/ml) | Angle of Repose | Compressibi-lity Index (%) | Drug Content (average)(%) |
|---|---|---|---|---|---|
| U-1 | 0.50 ± 0.03 | 0.59 ± 0.02 | 23.15±0.03 | 15.25 ±0.01 | 99.14 |
| U-2 | 0.47± 0.01 | 0.55 ± 0.03 | 23.05±0.01 | 14.55±0.02 | 99.67 |
| U-3 | 0.45± 0.04 | 0.56± 0.02 | 19.64±0.02 | 17.64±0.02 | 98.94 |
| M-1 | 0.47 ± 0.03 | 0.59 ± 0.05 | 21.25±0.04 | 20.34 ±0.04 | 99.54 |
| M-2 | 0.47 ± 0.01 | 0.57 ± 0.03 | 21.44±0.02 | 17.54 ±0.02 | 100.13 |
| M-3 | 0.49 ± 0.04 | 0.61 ± 0.02 | 22.53±0.01 | 19.67 ±0.03 | 99.98 |
| M-4 | 0.51 ± 0.04 | 0.62 ± 0.01 | 21.13±0. | 17.74 | 99.23 |

| | | | 04 | ±0.02 | |
|------|---------------|---------------|-----------|---------------|--------|
| M-5 | 0.49 ± 0.04 | 0.61 ± 0.03 | 22.43±0.03 | 17.39 ±0.04 | 100.21 |

NB: Sample tested from 5 point for each formulation

## 3.2 Evaluation of Tablet

The tablets of the proposed formulations (U-1 to U-3 and M-1 to M-5) were subjected to various evaluation tests like thickness, hardness, weight variation test and friability test, Drug content (Table 3.3).

### 3.2.1 Thickness

The thickness of the tablets for formulation U-1 to U-3 ranged from 6.50 ± 0.05 to 6.66 ± 0.07 and for formulation M-1 to M-5.

### 3.2.2 Hardness

Ten tablets of each of the formulations were taken and hardness was measured by Hardness tester (Sotax HT10, Switzerland).

**Table 3.2: Hardness of the formulation U-1 to U-3 and M-1 to M-5**

| Formulations | Hardness (Kp) |
|--------------|----------------|
| U-1 | 6.1 ± 0.15 |
| U-2 | 7.2 ± 0.13 |
| U-3 | 6.4 ± 0.17 |
| M-1 | 12.2 ± 0.11 |
| M-2 | 11.8 ± 0.16 |
| M-3 | 13.9 ± 0.15 |
| M-4 | 12.3 ± 0.14 |
| M-5 | 13.1 ± 0.14 |

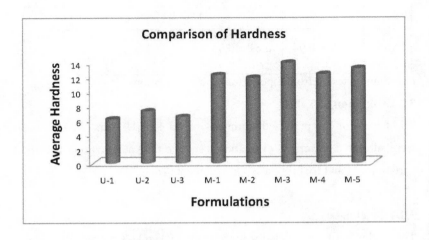

**Figure 3.1: Comparison of Hardness**

### 3.2.3 Friability

Friability of the tablet of proposed formulations were ranged from 0.20 ± 0.01% to 0.53 ± 0.02%.

### 3.2.4 Weight Variation

Weight variation of tablet in each formula were within pharmacopoeial limit and for formulation U-1 to U-3 were ranged from 1.08 ± 0.05% to 1.30 ± 0.02 and for formulation M-1 to M-5 were 1.15 ± 0.07% to 2.10 ± 0.03

### 3.2.5 Drug content

The drug content in a weighed amount of all formulations ranged from 98.00 ± 0.08 to 100.27 ± 0.04%.

**Table 3.3:** Properties of Metronidazole extended release tablet containing Eudragit NM30D and Methocel Premium K4M as release retardant.

| Formulations | Thickness (mm) | Weight Variation (%) | Drug Content (%) | Hardness (Kp) | Friability (%) |
|---|---|---|---|---|---|
| U-1 | 6.50 ± 0.05 | 1.12 ± 0.02 | 100.77±0.10 | 6.1 ± 0.15 | 0.50 ± 0.01 |
| U-2 | 6.66 ± 0.07 | 1.08 ± 0.05 | 99.93 ± 0.05 | 7.2 ± 0.13 | 0.53 ± 0.02 |
| U-3 | 6.53 ± 0.03 | 1.30 ± 0.02 | 99.09 ± 0.05 | 6.4 ± 0.17 | 0.33 ± 0.01 |
| M-1 | 6.95 ± 0.02 | 2.10 ± 0.03 | 100.67±0.05 | 12.2 ± 0.11 | 0.35 ± 0.03 |
| M-2 | 6.90 ± 0.01 | 1.25 ± 0.01 | 99.93 ± 0.03 | 11.8 ± 0.16 | 0.26 ± 0.02 |
| M-3 | 6.83 ± 0.03 | 1.23 ± 0.04 | 99.09 ± 0.01 | 13.9 ± 0.15 | 0.33 ± 0.01 |
| M-4 | 6.87 ± 0.06 | 1.17 ± 0.03 | 100.09±0.04 | 12.3 ± 0.14 | 0.20 ± 0.01 |
| M-5 | 6.93 ± 0.05 | 1.15 ± 0.07 | 99.09 ± 0.01 | 13.1 ± 0.14 | 0.48 ± 0.01 |

The average percentage of deviation of 10 tablets of each formula was less than ± 6%. Drug content among different batches of tablets ranged from 98.00 ± 0.08 to 100.27 ± 0.04%. In a weight variation test, the pharmacopeial limit for the percentage deviation for tablets was ± 0.5%. Good uniformity in drug content among different batches of the tablets was found and the percentage of drug content was more than 97%. In this study, the percentage friability for all the formulations was below 1%, indicating that the friability was within the official limits. All the tablet formulation showed acceptable pharmacopoeial properties and complied with the in-house specifications for weight variation, drug content, hardness and friability.

## 3.3 Dissolution

For the development of Metronidazole extended release dosage form and study of release profile with innovator drugs, Eudragit NM30D and Methocel Premium K4M were used separately as release retardant by wet granulation method. Three formulations were developed by using Eudragit NM30D and another five formulations were developed by using Methocel Premium K4M.

The objective of this study is to evaluate the comparative efficacy of abovementioned polymers on sustaining the release of Metronidazole. The effect of Eudragit NM30D and Methocel K4M on Metronidazole sustained release dosage was assessed.

Three formulations (U-1, U-2, U-3) containing Eudragit NM30D in amount of 9mg, 12mg and 15mg of per tablet were performed. Five of another formulations (M-1, M-2, M-3, M-4 and M-5) Methocel PremiumK4M in amount of 30mg, 35mg, 38.5mg, 40mg and 45mg per tablet were also performed.

The dissolution study of formulations (U-1, U-2, U-3 and M-1, M-2, M-3, M-4, M-5) Eudragit NM30D and Methocel K4M based tablet matrices were carried out in 0.1 N Hydrochloric acid for 12 hours period. The percent released of active from proposed formulations (U-1, U-2 and U-3) containing Eudragit NM30D based polymer matrices were summarized on the Table-3.4. The percent release of active from proposed formulations (M-1, M-2, M-3, M-4 and M-5) containing Methocel Premium K4M based polymer matrices are summarized on the Table 3.8.

### 3.3.1 Effect of polymeric content on the release profile of drugs

The effect of polymer content on drug-release as a function of time was found to be significantly different for a specific drug and polymer irrespective of chemical nature. Comparing the release profile for a particular polymer system from Figure 3.2 and Figure 3.6, it can be observed that, for the drug under investigation, drug release is inversely proportional to the level of rate retarding polymer present in the matrix system, i.e. the rate and extent of drug release increases with decrease in total polymeric content of the matrix. A linear relationship exist between the polymer content and rate of drug release irrespective of physico-chemical nature of drug and polymer as characterized by higher values of correlation-coefficient. This finding is in accordance with Reza *et al.*, 2002. The rate of drug release was calculated from the slope of the Higuchi curve expressed as % drug released vs square route of time. The decrease in the drug release rate with the increase in the polymer content due to a decrease in the total porosity of the matrices (initial porosity and porosity due to the dissolution of the drug) (Quadir *et al.*, 2002). Again, the reduced amount of drug retarding polymer was replaced by Lactose. Lactose caused a decrease in the tortuosity of the diffusion path of the drug (BASF, 1999).

Analogous result was reported with previous investigation (Kabir *et al.*, 2009).

### 3.3.2 Effect of polymer type on the release profile of drug

The release profile of active ingredient was influenced by the class and nature of matrix forming polymers. Types of polymers used to prepare the matrix were also found to impart differential effect on matrix disintegration. The effect of polymer type on drug-release as a function of time can be observed by comparing the corresponding release profile of drug from any matrix system at different polymeric level in Figure 3.2 and Figure 3.6. Drug release was higher from the matrices containing Methocel Premium K4M compared to Edragit NM30D. The fact can be described on the basis of polymeric nature and the mechanism by which the polymers release drug in the surrounding medium (Quadir *et al.*, 2003). Eudragit NM30D is a pH-independent polymethacrylate copolymer dispersion which is potentially erodible and controls the release of drug through pore diffusion and erosion mechanism.

The ability of Methocel Premium K4M to retard the drug release by swelling in aqueous media is also reported. (Michailova *et al.*, 2000). The ability of a polymer to retard drug release rate is related to its viscosity. However, processing factors including particle size, hardness, porosity and compressibility index also affect the release rate of drug from the tablet. Different grades of HPMC are available depending on their hydration rate which in turns depends on the nature of substituent like Hydroxypropyl group content. (Kabir *et al.*, 2009). Methocel Premium K4M was used for this model as it forms a strong viscous gel in contact with aqueous media, which may be useful in controlled drug delivery. This finding is carried out in accordance with the work carried out by (Hogan, 1989).

### 3.3.3 Release Kinetics

The drug release data obtained were extrapolated by Zero Order, First Order, Higuchi and Korsmeyer-Peppas, and model independent Difference factor and Similarity factor equation to know the mechanism of drug release from these formulations (Higuchi, 1961 and Korsmeyer *et al.*,1983). In this study, the in *vitro* release profiles of drugs from the formulations U-1 to U-3 could be best expressed by First Order equation, as the plot shows highest linearity ( $R^2$ : 0.994 to 0.931 ). Finally, the release rate of these three formulations U-1 to F-3 were compared with the innovator's drug Flagyl ER Tablet in terms of Difference Factor ($f_1$) and Similarity Factor ($f_2$ ) (Table 3.14- 3.16) (Laila *et al.*, 2009). But among these three formulations U-3 was not bioequivalent with the Innovator drug compared to Difference Factor ($f_1$) and similarity factor $f_2$ (Flagyl ER Tablet).

At the same time among the proposed formulations M-1 to M-5 formulation M-3 showed desired dissolution pattern. Release profile of M-4 was also quite satisfactory. The fractional release profiles of Metronidazole versus time over 12 hours matrix with different contents of Methocel Premium K4M (M-1 to M-5 Table 3.8-3.11) are shown in (Fig.3.6 to 3.9). Since Methocel Premium K4M is the rate-controlling agent, an increase in the content of Methocel Premium K4M in the matrix causes a decrease in the fractional release. In this study, the in *vitro* release profiles of drugs from the formulations M-1 to M-5 3 could be best

123

expressed by First Order equation, as the plot shows highest linearity ( $R^2$ : 0.996 to 0.910 ).

The dissolution profiles of proposed formulations M-1 to M-5 were compared with Innovator drug in term of Difference Factor ($f_1$) and Similarity factor ($f_2$). It was observed that formulation M-3 showed the highest similarity and lowest difference factor with the innovators' drug Flagyl ER Tablet i.e. it is bioequivalent with the innovator drugs. Proposed formulation M-1 and M-5 were not bioequivalent with the innovator drug in term Difference Factor ($f_1$) and Similarity factor ($f_2$). Formulations U-2, M-3 and M-4 showed better dissolution rate than other proposed formulations. But the hardness of all the formulation using Eudragit NM30D as release retardant was to poor to blister packing for commercialization. Considering all factors proposed formulation M-3 was selected as suitable candidate for Stability study.

## 3.4 Effect of Eudragit NM30D on release pattern of Metronidazole BP from matrix tablet

Different Eudragit NM30D matrix tablet containing Metronidazole BP as active ingredient having Eudragit NM30D polymer 9 mg, 12 mg and 15 mg per tablet in the matrix tablet with the formulation code U-1, U-2 and U-3were prepared by direct compression to evaluate the effect of this polymer and granulation process. After preparation according to formulation shown in the Table 2.4, their dissolution studies were carried out in paddle method (USP-II) with a sinker at 100 rpm in phosphate buffer medium at $37^0$ c ($\pm 0.5^0$c). Six tablets from each formulation were used in dissolution study. The release profile of Metronidazoleb was monitored up to 12 hours. The average release pattern is shown in Figure 3.2. Figure 3.4

represents the Higuchi impact that is obtained by plotting the % of drug release vs Square Root of Time (SQRT). First order release pattern has been shown in Figure 3.3. Korsmeyer release pattern has been obtained by plotting log cumulative percent drug release vs log time (Figure 3.5). The percent of drug release from these three formulations at different time intervals are shown at the Table 3.4.

A release profile of Metrronidazole containing Eudragit NM30D matrix tablet compressed by wet granulation for three formulations was obtained from the graphs. The total % of Metronidazole release from the formulation U-1, U-2 and U-3 was 98.63% 94.12% and 77.56% respectively. It has been observed that the release rate has been extended with the increase of polymer % and with the decrease of lactose %. The highest percent of drug release within 12 hours is obtained from U-1 where polymer content is 9 mg tablet. But in U-3, the polymer content is 15 mg per tablet and the release of drug is controlled with 77.56% within 12 hours.

The rate of drug release was found to be inversely related to the amount of Eudragit NM30D present in the matrix structure, i.e. the drug release increased with decrease in the polymer content of the matrix tablet. Such increase in polymer content results in a decrease in the drug release rate due to a decrease in the total porosity i.e. release is extended to long period. Lactose causes a decreased tortuosity of the path of the drug due to its preferential solubility than Eudragit NM30D, by its swelling effect, additionally weakened the integrity of the matrix (Nixon, Patel and Tong, 1995).

**Table 3.4:** Zero order release profile Eudragit NM30D based Metronidazole Matrix Tablets

| Time | U-1 | U-2 | U-3 |
|------|-------|-------|-------|
| 0 | 0.00 | 0.00 | 0.00 |
| 1 | 20.15 | 16.47 | 12.11 |
| 2 | 46.10 | 38.12 | 29.89 |
| 4 | 68.33 | 61.23 | 41.73 |
| 6 | 91.91 | 74.19 | 59.68 |
| 8 | 98.61 | 81.23 | 67.19 |
| 10 | 98.86 | 88.89 | 73.11 |
| 12 | 98.63 | 94.12 | 77.56 |

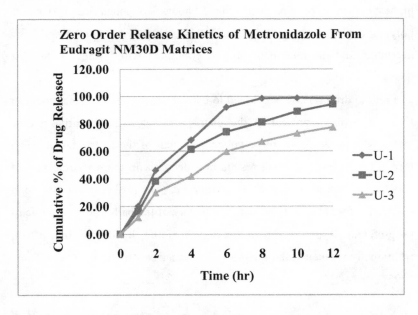

**Figure 3.2:** Zero order plot of release kinetics of Metronidazole from Eudragit NM30D Matrices

**Table 3.5: First order release profile Eudragit NM30D based Metronidazole Matrix Tablets**

| Time (hrs) | U-1 | U-2 | U-3 |
|------------|-----------|----------|----------|
| 0 | 2 | 2 | 2 |
| 1 | 1.902275 | 1.921842 | 1.943939 |
| 2 | 1.731589 | 1.79155 | 1.84578 |
| 4 | 1.500648 | 1.588496 | 1.765445 |
| 6 | 0.907949 | 1.411788 | 1.605521 |
| 8 | 0.143015 | 1.273464 | 1.516006 |
| 10 | 0.056905 | 1.045714 | 1.429591 |
| 12 | 0.136721 | 0.769377 | 1.351023 |

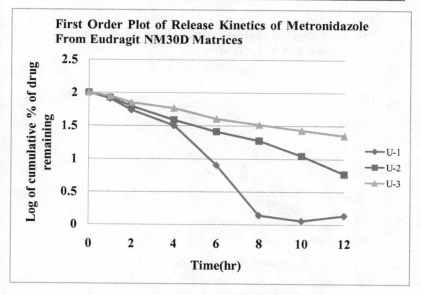

Figure 3.3: First order plot of release kinetics of Metronidazole from Eudragit NM30D Matrices

**Table 3.6: Higuchi release profile Eudragit NM30D based Metronidazole Matrix Tablets**

| SQRT | U-1 | U-2 | U-3 |
|------|------|------|------|
| 0.00 | 0.00 | 0.00 | 0.00 |
| 1.00 | 20.15 | 16.47 | 12.11 |
| 1.41 | 46.10 | 38.12 | 29.89 |
| 2.00 | 68.33 | 61.23 | 41.73 |
| 2.45 | 91.91 | 74.19 | 59.68 |
| 2.83 | 98.61 | 81.23 | 67.19 |
| 3.16 | 98.86 | 88.89 | 73.11 |
| 3.46 | 98.63 | 94.12 | 77.56 |

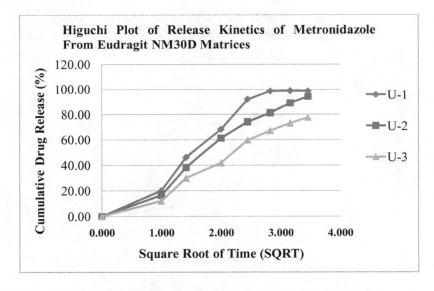

**Figure 3.4: Higuchi plot of release kinetics of Metronidazole from Eudragit NM30D Matrices**

**Table 3.7: Korsmeyer release profile Eudragit NM30D based Metronidazole Matrix Tablets**

| Log of Time | U-1 | U-2 | U-3 |
|:---:|:---:|:---:|:---:|
| 0.00000 | 1.30428 | 1.21669 | 1.08314 |
| 0.30103 | 1.66370 | 1.58115 | 1.47553 |
| 0.60206 | 1.83461 | 1.78696 | 1.62045 |
| 0.77815 | 1.96336 | 1.87035 | 1.77583 |
| 0.90309 | 1.99392 | 1.90972 | 1.82730 |
| 1.00000 | 1.99502 | 1.94885 | 1.86398 |
| 1.07918 | 1.99401 | 1.97368 | 1.88964 |

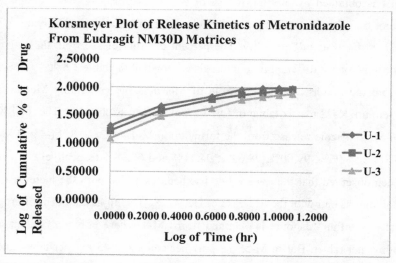

**Figure 3.5: Korsmeyer plot of release kinetics of Metronidazole from Eudragit NM30D Matrices**

## 3.5 Effect of Methocel Premium K4M on release pattern of Metrnidazole from matrix tablet by wet granulation

For this experiment, different Methocel PremiumK4M matrix tablet containing Metrnidazole as active ingredient having Methocel PremiumK4M polymer 30 mg, 35 mg, 38.5mg , 40 mg and 45 mg per 1100 mg tablet weight in the matrix tablet with the formulation code M-1, M-2, M-3, M-4 and M-5 were prepared. After preparation according to formulation shown in the Table 2.8, their dissolution studies were carried out in paddle method (USP-II) with a sinker at 100 rpm in 0.1N Hydrochloric Acid medium at $37^0$ c ($\pm 0.5^0$c). Six tablets from each formulation were used in dissolution study. The release profile of Metronidazole was monitored up to 12 hours. The zero order release pattern is shown in figure 3.6. Figure 3.8 represents the Higuchi impact that is obtained by plotting the % of cumulative drug release vs Square Root of Time (SQRT). First order release profile is shown in Figure 3.7 and Korsmeyer in Figure 3.9. The percent of drug release from these five formulations at different time intervals is shown at the table 3.8

From the graphs, a release profile of Metrnidazole containing Methocel Premium K4M matrix tablet of five formulations was obtained. The total % of Metrnidazole release from the formulation M-1, M-2, M-3, M-4 and M-5 were 98.96%, 99.00%, 98.63%, 94.11% and 60.98% respectively. It has been observed that the release rate has been extended with the increase of polymer % and with the decrease of lactose %. The highest percent of drug release within 12 hours is obtained from M-1 where polymer content is 30mg per tablet. But in M-5, the polymer content is 45 mg per tablet and the release of drug is controlled with 60.98% within 12 hours. For this further increase of polymer percentage was not done.

The rate of drug release was found to be inversely related to the amount of Methocel Premium K4M present in the matrix structure, i.e. the drug release increased with decrease in the polymer content of the matrix tablet.

Such increase in polymer content results in a decrease in the drug release rate due to a decrease in the total porosity i.e. release is extended to long period. Lactose causes a decreased tortuosity of the path of the drug due to its preferential solubility than Methocel Premium K4M, by its swelling effect, additionally weakened the integrity of the matrix (Nixon, Patel and Tong, 1995)

**Table 3.8: Zero order release profile Methocel Premium K4M based Metronidazole Matrix Tablets**

| Time | M-1 | M-2 | M-3 | M-4 | M-5 |
|------|------|------|------|------|------|
| 0 | 0.00 | 0.00 | 0.00 | 0.00 | 0.00 |
| 1 | 26.30 | 18.13 | 14.76 | 12.29 | 11.88 |
| 2 | 52.50 | 46.15 | 40.86 | 35.45 | 27.21 |
| 4 | 81.10 | 70.49 | 64.93 | 53.55 | 43.10 |
| 6 | 96.32 | 91.22 | 83.54 | 72.10 | 52.19 |
| 8 | 98.82 | 98.11 | 92.11 | 83.66 | 56.20 |
| 10 | 98.78 | 98.94 | 97.89 | 90.12 | 58.17 |
| 12 | 98.96 | 99.00 | 98.63 | 94.11 | 60.98 |

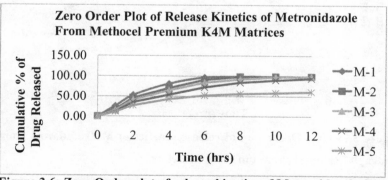

Figure 3.6: Zero Order plot of release kinetics of Metronidazole from Eudragit Methocel Premium K4M Matrices

131

**Table 3.9: First order release profile Methocel Premium K4M based Metronidazole Matrix Tablets**

| Time | M-1 | M-2 | M-3 | M-4 | M-5 |
|------|------|------|------|------|------|
| 0 | 2 | 2 | 2 | 2 | 2 |
| 1 | 1.867467 | 1.913125 | 1.930643 | 1.943049 | 1.945074 |
| 2 | 1.676694 | 1.731186 | 1.771881 | 1.809896 | 1.862072 |
| 4 | 1.276462 | 1.469969 | 1.544936 | 1.666986 | 1.755112 |
| 6 | 0.565848 | 0.943495 | 1.21643 | 1.445604 | 1.679519 |
| 8 | 0.071882 | 0.276462 | 0.897077 | 1.213252 | 1.641474 |
| 10 | 0.08636 | 0.025306 | 0.324282 | 0.994757 | 1.621488 |
| 12 | 0.017033 | 0 | 0.136721 | 0.770115 | 1.591287 |

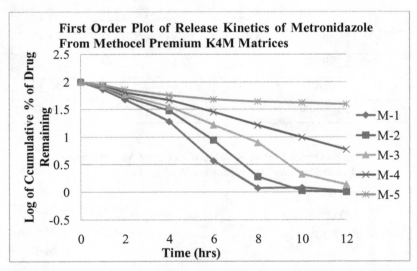

**Figure 3.7: First Order plot of release kinetics of Metronidazole from Eudragit Methocel Premium K4M Matrices**

**Table 3.10: Higuchi release profile Methocel Premium K4M based Metronidazole Matrix Tablets**

| SQRT | M-1 | M-2 | M-3 | M-4 | M-5 |
|------|------|------|------|------|------|
| 0.00 | 0.00 | 0.00 | 0.00 | 0.00 | 0.00 |
| 1.00 | 26.30 | 18.13 | 14.76 | 12.29 | 11.88 |
| 1.41 | 52.50 | 46.15 | 40.86 | 35.45 | 27.21 |
| 2.00 | 81.10 | 70.49 | 64.93 | 53.55 | 43.10 |
| 2.45 | 96.32 | 91.22 | 83.54 | 72.10 | 52.19 |
| 2.83 | 98.82 | 98.11 | 92.11 | 83.66 | 56.20 |
| 3.16 | 98.78 | 98.94 | 97.89 | 90.12 | 58.17 |
| 3.46 | 98.96 | 99.00 | 98.63 | 94.11 | 60.98 |

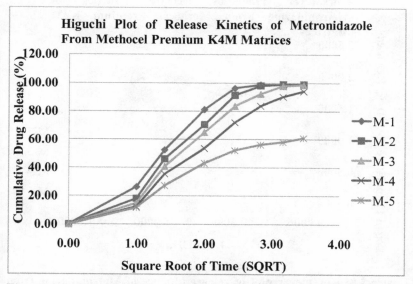

Figure 3.8: Higuchi plot of release kinetics of Metronidazole from Eudragit Methocel Premium K4M Matrices

**Table 3.11: Korsmeyer release profile Methocel Premium K4M based Metronidazole Matrix Tablets**

| Log of Time | M-1 | M-2 | M-3 | M-4 | M-5 |
|---|---|---|---|---|---|
| 0.0000 | 1.4200 | 1.2584 | 1.1691 | 1.0896 | 1.0748 |
| 0.3010 | 1.7202 | 1.6642 | 1.6113 | 1.5496 | 1.4347 |
| 0.6021 | 1.9090 | 1.8481 | 1.8124 | 1.7288 | 1.6345 |
| 0.7782 | 1.9837 | 1.9601 | 1.9219 | 1.8579 | 1.7176 |
| 0.9031 | 1.9948 | 1.9917 | 1.9643 | 1.9225 | 1.7497 |
| 1.0000 | 1.9947 | 1.9954 | 1.9907 | 1.9548 | 1.7647 |
| 1.0792 | 1.9955 | 1.9956 | 1.9940 | 1.9736 | 1.7852 |

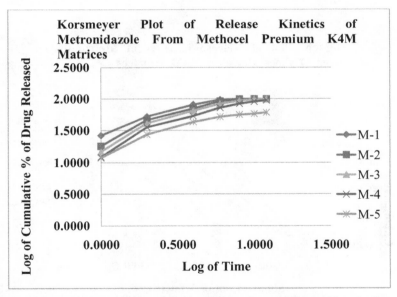

**Figure 3.9: Korsmeyer plot of release kinetics of Metronidazole from Eudragit Methocel Premium K4M Matrices**

**3.6  Determination of release Kinetics from multiple co-efficient**

134

The drug release data from the proposed formulations U-1 to U-3 were treated in different kinetics order (Zero order plot, First order, Higuchi plot and Korsmeyer) and their correlation coefficients were determined graphically to identify their release mechanism. The drug percent release was plotted against time to get zero order release kinetics, Log % drug remaining against time to get first order release kinetics, percent release versus square root of time to get Higuchi release kinetics and percent release versus log of time to get korsmeyer release kinetics. From correlation coefficient it can be determined the mechanism of release kinetics. The correlation coefficient getting close to 1.0, the release kinetics will be followed that order of proposed formulations. The correlation coefficients were determined graphically (shown in Fig: 3.10 to 3.21).

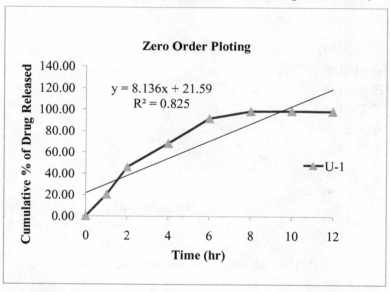

**Figure: 3.10: Zero Order plot of the proposed formulation (U-1)**

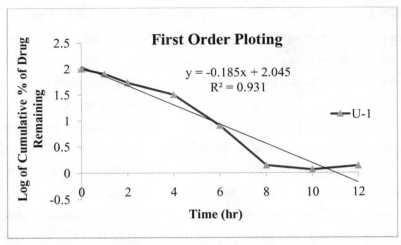

**Figure: 3.11: First Order plot of the proposed formulation (U-1)**

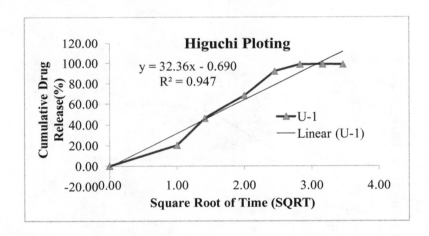

**Figure: 3.12: Higuchi plot of the proposed formulation (U-1)**

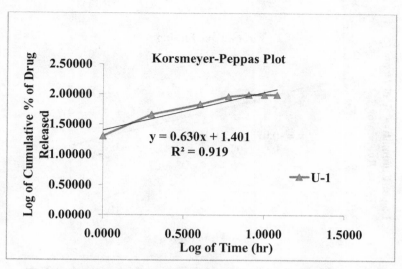

Figure: 3.13: Korsmeyer plot of the proposed formulation (U-1)

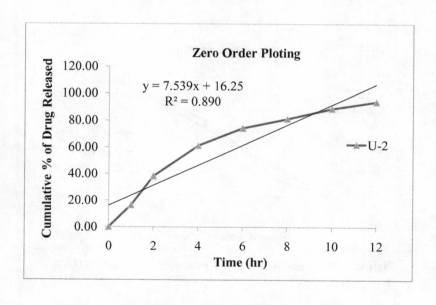

Figure: 3.14: Zero Order plot of the proposed formulation (U-2)

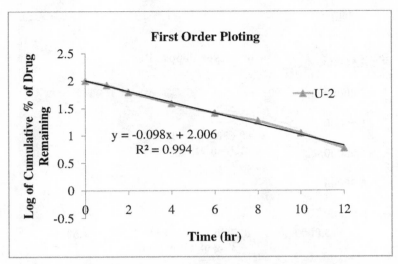

**Figure: 3.15: First Order plot of the proposed formulation (U-2)**

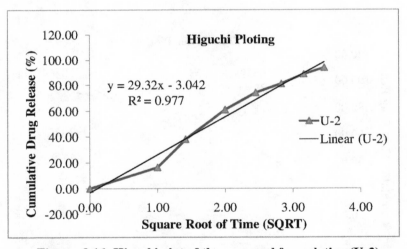

**Figure: 3.16: Higuchi plot of the proposed formulation (U-2)**

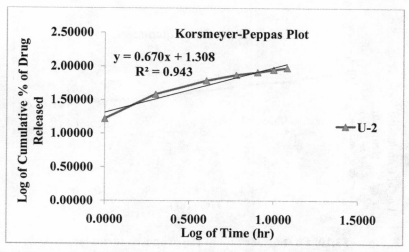

Figure: 3.17: Korsmeyer plot of the proposed formulation (U-2)

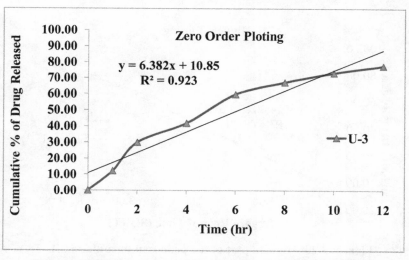

Figure: 3.18: Zero Order plot of the proposed formulation (U-3)

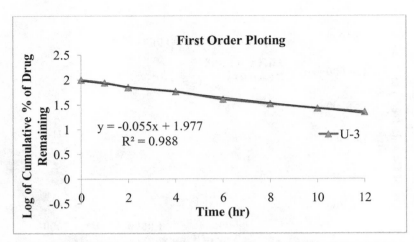

Figure: 3.19: First Order plot of the proposed formulation (U-3)

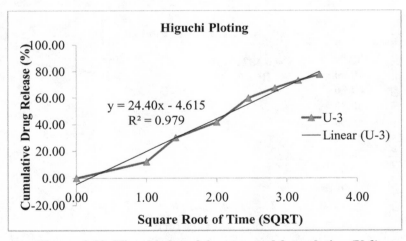

Figure: 3.20: Higuchi plot of the proposed formulation (U-3)

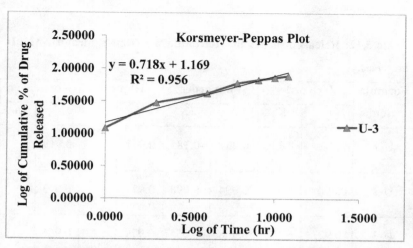

**Figure: 3.21: Korsmeyer plot of the proposed formulation (U-3)**

The release kinetics data has been mention in the Table 3.12. From the table it has been seen that all these formulations of this class show good linearity for First order plot ($r^2$ : 0.931, 0.994 and 0.988). Good linearity also shown for Korsmeyer plot ($r^2$ : 0.919, 0.943 and 0.956) where the formulations follow Anomalous / non – Fickian transport (n: >0.45 or < 0.89). From the table it has been seen that all these formulations of this class follows zero order Korsmeyer and Higuchi release model. Formulation U-2 to U-3 best fit with First order release model followed by Higuchi, Korsmeyer and zero order

**Table 3.12: Release kinetics of Metronidazole from Eudragit NM30D matrices.**

| Formulation | Zero order | | First order | | Higuchi | | Korsmeyer | |
|---|---|---|---|---|---|---|---|---|
| | $r^2$ | $K_0$ | $r^2$ | $K_1$ | $r^2$ | $K_H$ | $r^2$ | n |
| U-1 | 0.825 | 8.136 | 0.931 | -0.185 | 0.947 | 32.36 | 0.919 | 0.630 |
| U-2 | 0.890 | 7.539 | 0.994 | -0.098 | 0.977 | 29.32 | 0.943 | 0.670 |
| U-3 | 0.923 | 6.382 | 0.988 | -0.055 | 0.979 | 24.40 | 0.956 | 0.718 |

Likewise formulations U-1 to U-3, M-1 to M-5 were treated in different kinetics order (Zero order plot, First order plot and Higuchi plot) and their correlation coefficients were determined graphically to identify their release mechanism. The correlation coefficients were determined graphically (shown in Fig: 3.22 to 3.41).

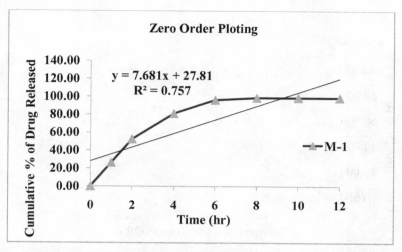

Figure: 3.22: Zero Order plot of the proposed formulation (M-1)

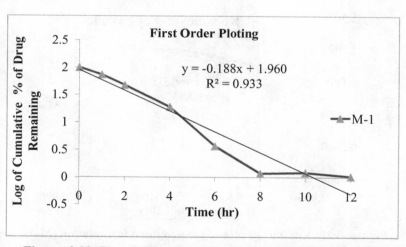

Figure: 3.23: First Order plot of the proposed formulation (M-1)

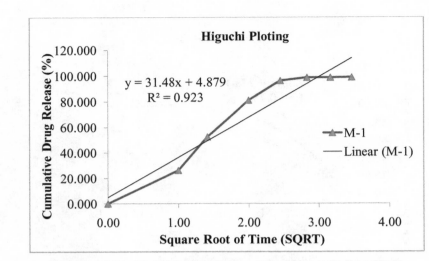

**Figure: 3.24: Higuchi plot of the proposed formulation (M-1)**

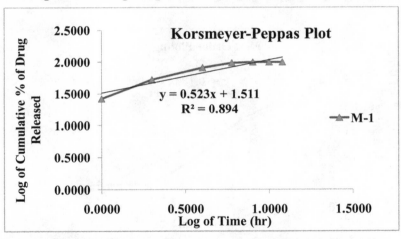

**Figure: 3.25: Korsmeyer plot of the proposed formulation (M-1)**

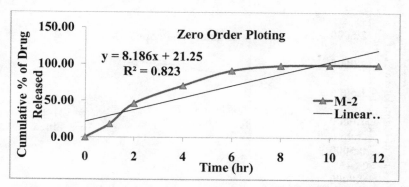

**Figure: 3.26: Zero Order plot of the proposed formulation (M-2)**

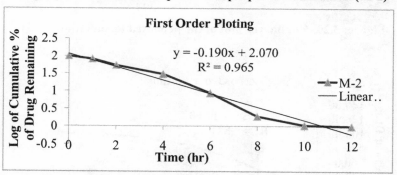

**Figure: 3.27: First Order plot of the proposed formulation (M-2)**

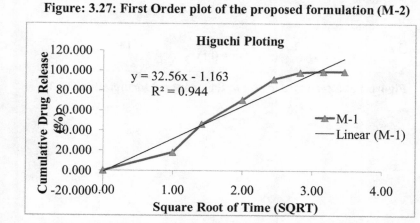

**Figure: 3.28: Higuchi plot of the proposed formulation (M-2)**

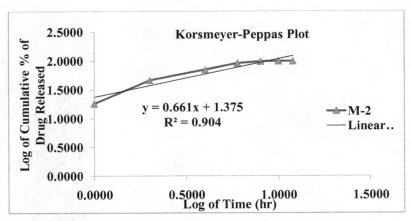

Figure: 3.29: Korsmeyer plot of the proposed formulation (M-2)

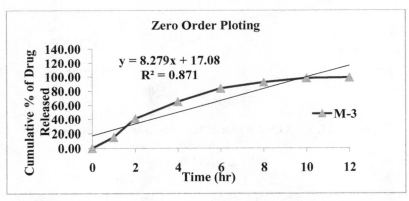

Figure 3.30: Zero Order plot of the proposed formulation (M-3)

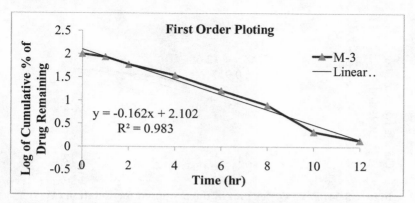

**Figure 3.31: First Order plot of the proposed formulation (M-3)**

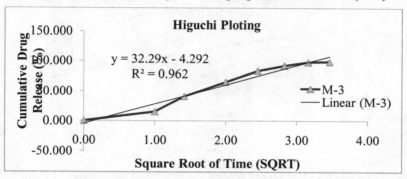

**Figure 3.32: Higuchi plot of the proposed formulation (M-3)**

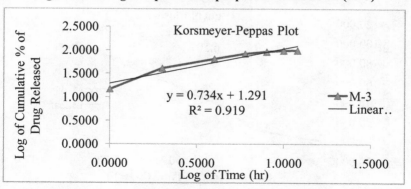

**Figure 3.33: Korsmeyer plot of the proposed formulation (M-3)**

147

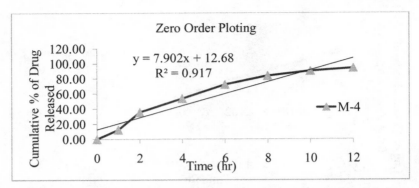

**Figure 3.34: Zero Order plot of the proposed formulation (M-4)**

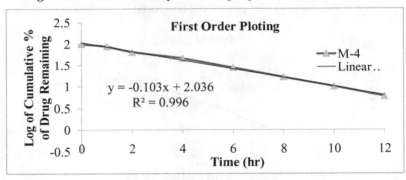

**Figure 3.35: First Order plot of the proposed formulation (M-4)**

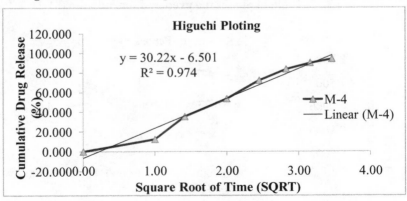

**Figure 3.36: Higuchi plot of the proposed formulation (M-4)**

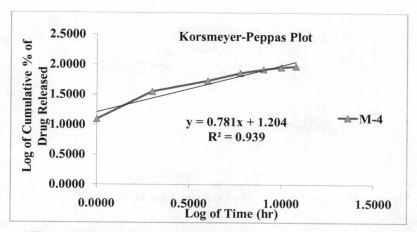

**Figure 3.37: Korsmeyer plot of the proposed formulation (M-4)**

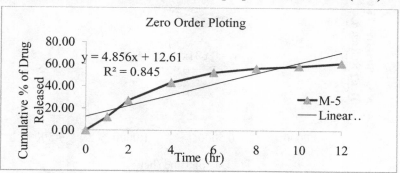

**Figure 3.38: Zero Order plot of the proposed formulation (M-5)**

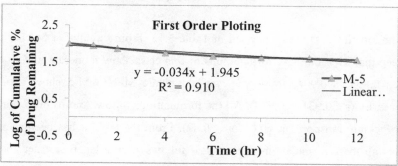

**Figure 3.39: First Order plot of the proposed formulation (M-5)**

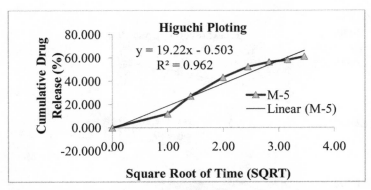

**Figure 3.40: Higuchi plot of the proposed formulation (M-5)**

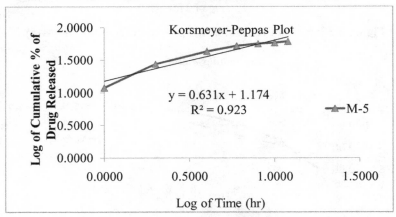

**Figure 3.41: Korsmeyer plot of the proposed formulation (M-5)**

The kinetics data are mentioned in Table 3.13. From the table it has been seen that M-1 and M-2 formulations of this class show moderate linearity ($r^2$: 0.894 to 0.904) for Korsmeyer plot while M-3 to M-5 show good linearity ($r^2$ : 0.931 to 0.919). All the formulations follow Anomalous / non – Fickian transport (n: >0.45 or < 0.89). From the table it has been seen that all these formulations of this class follows zero order, first order and Higuchi release model. Formulation M-2, M-3 and M-4 best fit with first order release model follow by Higuchi and zero order where M-5 best fit for Higuchi release profile.

**Table 3.13: Release kinetics of Metronidazole from Methocel Premium K4M matrices.**

| Formulation | Zero order | | First order | | Higuchi | | Korsmeyer | |
|---|---|---|---|---|---|---|---|---|
| | $r^2$ | $K_0$ | $r^2$ | $K_1$ | $r^2$ | $K_H$ | $r^2$ | n |
| M-1 | 0.757 | 7.681 | 0.933 | -0.188 | 0.923 | 31.48 | 0.894 | 0.532 |
| M-2 | 0.823 | 8.186 | 0.965 | -0.190 | 0.944 | 32.56 | 0.904 | 0.661 |
| M-3 | 0.871 | 8.279 | 0.983 | -0.162 | 0.962 | 32.29 | 0.919 | 0.734 |
| M-4 | 0.917 | 7.902 | 0.996 | -0.103 | 0.974 | 30.22 | 0.931 | 0.781 |
| M-5 | 0.845 | 4.856 | 0.910 | -0.034 | 0.962 | 19.22 | 0.923 | 0.631 |

### 3.7 Bioequivalence Study

The release rate of formulations were compared with the innovator's drug Flagyl ER Tablet in terms of Difference Factor ($f_1$) and Similarity Factor ($f_2$) (Table 3.14.- 3.20) (Laila *et al.*, 2009).For this purpose **Flagyl ER** worldwide brand product of **Pfizer**, was collected from market and dissolution of this was studied for 12 hours in the same condition of the test sample. Here the release of Flagyl ER treated as reference standard. Difference Factor ($f_1$) and Similarity Factor ($f_2$) are summarized in Table 3.21.

Here to compare the release kinetics of proposed Metronidazole ER Tablets with the Innovator's drug Flagyl ER tablet approaches were used including model independent method of the difference factor ($f_1$) and similarity factor ($f_2$).

**Table 3.14: Difference and Similarity factor of release pattern between Flagyl ER Tablet and proposed formulation U-1.**

| U-1 | | | | |
|---|---|---|---|---|
| Time | $R_t$ | $T_t$ | $[R_t\text{-}T_t]$ | $(R_t\text{-}T_t)^2$ |
| 1 | 16.17 | 20.15 | 3.98 | 15.8404 |
| 2 | 39.93 | 46.10 | 6.17 | 38.0689 |
| 4 | 63.92 | 68.33 | 4.41 | 19.4481 |
| 6 | 79.87 | 91.91 | 12.04 | 144.9616 |
| 8 | 88.25 | 98.61 | 10.36 | 107.3296 |
| 10 | 91.91 | 98.86 | 6.95 | 48.3025 |
| 12 | 94.89 | 98.63 | 3.74 | 13.9876 |
| Total | 474.94 | 522.59 | 47.65 | 387.9387 |

$$f_1 = \frac{\sum [R_t - T_t]}{\sum R_t} \times 100$$

$f_1 =$ **10.03**      **[ NMT 15]**

$$(f_2) = 50 \log \{[1 + (1/N) \sum (R_t\text{-}T_t)]^{-0.5} \times 100\}$$

$f_2$  =  **56.21**      **[ NLT 50]**

Here,

$R_t$ = Percent dissolved for the reference standard at each time period.

$T_t$ = Percent dissolved for the test product at the same time period.

n = Number of time points in the dissolution profile.

$f_1$ = Difference factor to evaluate the equivalency of two products.

$f_2$ = Similarity factor to evaluate the equivalency of two products.

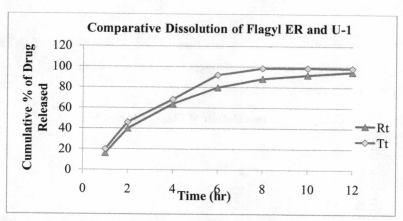

Figure 3.42: Comparative *in vitro* Metronidazole release profile for $f_1$ and $f_2$ test: Reference is Flagyl ER tablet and test is prepared U-1

Table 3.15: Difference and Similarity factor of release pattern between Flagyl ER Tablet and proposed formulation U-2.

| U-2 | | | | |
|---|---|---|---|---|
| Time | $R_t$ | $T_t$ | $[R_t-T_t]$ | $(R_t-T_t)^2$ |
| 1 | 16.17 | 16.47 | 0.30 | 0.09 |
| 2 | 39.93 | 38.12 | 1.81 | 3.2761 |
| 4 | 63.92 | 61.23 | 2.69 | 7.2361 |
| 6 | 79.87 | 74.19 | 5.68 | 32.2624 |
| 8 | 88.25 | 81.23 | 7.02 | 49.2804 |
| 10 | 91.91 | 88.89 | 3.02 | 9.1204 |
| 12 | 94.89 | 94.12 | 0.77 | 0.5929 |
| Total | 474.94 | 454.25 | 21.29 | 101.8583 |

$f_1 = 4.48$     [NMT 15]

$f_2 = 70.21$     [NLT 50]

Here difference factor $f_1$ is far less than 15 and similarity factor $f_2$ is far greater than 50 which indicate that test formulation U-2 and Flagyl ER has very similar release pattern

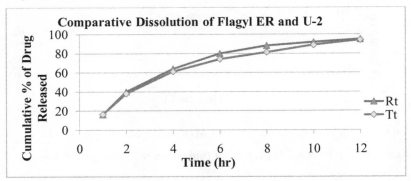

**Figure 3.43: Comparative *in vitro* Metronidazole release profile for $f_1$ and $f_2$ test: Reference is Flagyl ER tablet and test is prepared U-2.**

**Table 3.16: Difference and Similarity factor of release pattern between Flagyl ER Tablet and proposed formulation U-3.**

| U-3 | | | | |
|---|---|---|---|---|
| Time | $R_t$ | $T_t$ | $[R_t-T_t]$ | $(R_t-T_t)^2$ |
| 1 | 16.17 | 12.11 | 4.06 | 16.4836 |
| 2 | 39.93 | 29.89 | 10.04 | 100.8016 |
| 4 | 63.92 | 41.73 | 22.19 | 492.3961 |
| 6 | 79.87 | 59.68 | 20.19 | 407.6361 |
| 8 | 88.25 | 67.19 | 21.06 | 443.5236 |
| 10 | 91.91 | 73.11 | 18.80 | 353.44 |
| 12 | 94.89 | 77.56 | 17.33 | 300.3289 |
| **Total** | **474.94** | **361.27** | **113.67** | **2114.61** |

$f_1 = 23.93$    [ NMT 15 ]

$f_2 = 37.96$    [NLT 50]

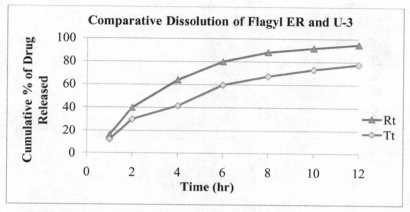

Figure 3.44: Comparative *in vitro* Metronidazole release profile for $f_1$ and $f_2$ test: Reference is Flagyl ER tablet and test is prepared U-3

Table 3.17: Difference and Similarity factor of release pattern between Flagyl ER Tablet and proposed formulation M-1.

| M-1 | | | | |
|---|---|---|---|---|
| Time | $R_t$ | $T_t$ | $[R_t-T_t]$ | $(R_t-T_t)^2$ |
| 1 | 16.17 | 26.30 | 10.13 | 102.6169 |
| 2 | 39.93 | 52.50 | 12.57 | 158.0049 |
| 4 | 63.92 | 81.10 | 17.18 | 295.1524 |
| 6 | 79.87 | 96.32 | 16.45 | 270.6025 |
| 8 | 88.25 | 98.82 | 10.57 | 111.7249 |
| 10 | 91.91 | 98.78 | 6.87 | 47.1969 |
| 12 | 94.89 | 98.96 | 4.07 | 16.5649 |
| Total | 474.94 | 552.78 | 77.84 | 1001.863 |

$f_1 = 16.38$    [NMT 15]

$f_2 = 46.03$    [NLT 50]

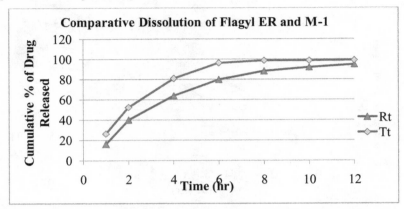

**Figure 3.45:** Comparative *in vitro* Metronidazole release profile for $f_1$ and $f_2$ test: Reference is Flagyl ER tablet and test is prepared M-1

**Table 3.18:** Difference and Similarity factor of release pattern between Flagyl ER Tablet and proposed formulation M-1.

| M-2 | | | | |
|---|---|---|---|---|
| Time | $R_t$ | $T_t$ | $[R_t\text{-}T_t]$ | $(R_t\text{-}T_t)^2$ |
| 1 | 16.17 | 18.13 | 1.96 | 3.8416 |
| 2 | 39.93 | 46.15 | 6.22 | 38.6884 |
| 4 | 63.92 | 70.49 | 6.57 | 43.1649 |
| 6 | 79.87 | 91.22 | 11.35 | 128.8225 |
| 8 | 88.25 | 98.11 | 9.86 | 97.2196 |
| 10 | 91.91 | 98.94 | 7.03 | 49.4209 |
| 12 | 94.89 | 99.00 | 4.11 | 16.8921 |
| Total | 474.94 | 522.04 | 47.1 | 378.05 |

$f_1 = 9.92$    [ NMT 15 ]; $f_2 = 56.49$    [NLT 50]

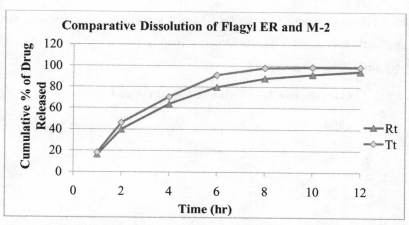

Figure 3.46: Comparative *in vitro* Metronidazole release profile for $f_1$ and $f_2$ test: Reference is Flagyl ER tablet and test is prepared M-2

Table 3.19: Difference and Similarity factor of release pattern between Flagyl ER Tablet and proposed formulation M-3.

| Time | $R_t$ | $T_t$ | $[R_t\text{-}T_t]$ | $(R_t\text{-}T_t)^2$ |
|------|-------|-------|--------|----------|
| M-3 | | | | |
| 1 | 16.17 | 14.76 | 1.41 | 1.9881 |
| 2 | 39.93 | 40.86 | 0.93 | 0.8649 |
| 4 | 63.92 | 64.93 | 1.01 | 1.0201 |
| 6 | 79.87 | 83.54 | 3.67 | 13.4689 |
| 8 | 88.25 | 92.11 | 3.86 | 14.8996 |
| 10 | 91.91 | 97.89 | 5.98 | 35.7604 |
| 12 | 94.89 | 98.63 | 3.74 | 13.9876 |
| Total | 474.94 | 492.72 | 20.6 | 81.9896 |

$f_1 = 4.34$     [NMT 15]; $f_2 = 72.39$     [NLT 50]

Here difference factor $f_1$ is far less than 15 and similarity factor $f_2$ is far greater than 50 which indicate that test formulation M-3 and Flagyl ER has very similar release pattern.

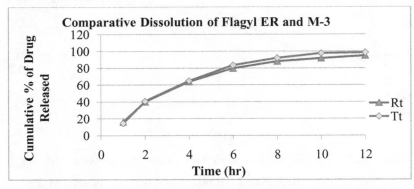

Fig 3.47: Comparative *in vitro* Metronidazole release profile for $f_1$ and $f_2$ test: Reference is Flagyl ER tablet and test is prepared M-3

Table 3.20: Difference and Similarity factor of release pattern between Flagyl ER Tablet and proposed formulation M-4.

| M-4 | | | | |
|---|---|---|---|---|
| Time | $R_t$ | $T_t$ | $[R_t-T_t]$ | $(R_t-T_t)^2$ |
| 1 | 16.17 | 12.29 | 3.88 | 15.0544 |
| 2 | 39.93 | 35.45 | 4.48 | 20.0704 |
| 4 | 63.92 | 53.55 | 10.37 | 107.5369 |
| 6 | 79.87 | 72.10 | 7.77 | 60.3729 |
| 8 | 88.25 | 83.66 | 4.59 | 21.0681 |
| 10 | 91.91 | 90.12 | 1.79 | 3.2041 |
| 12 | 94.89 | 94.11 | 0.78 | 0.6084 |
| Total | 474.94 | 441.28 | 33.66 | 227.9152 |

$f_1 = 7.08$      [NMT 15]; $f_2 = 61.85$      [NLT 50]

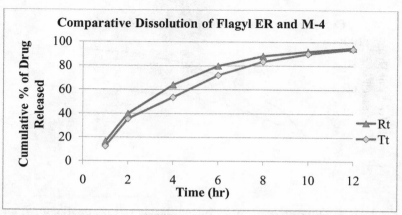

Fig 3.48: Comparative *in vitro* Metronidazole release profile for $f_1$ and $f_2$ test: Reference is Flagyl ER tablet and test is prepared M-4

Table 3.21: Difference and Similarity factor of release pattern between Flagyl ER Tablet and proposed formulation M-5.

| M-5 | | | | |
|---|---|---|---|---|
| Time | $R_t$ | $T_t$ | $[R_t-T_t]$ | $(R_t-T_t)^2$ |
| 1 | 16.17 | 11.88 | 4.29 | 18.4041 |
| 2 | 39.93 | 27.21 | 12.72 | 161.7984 |
| 4 | 63.92 | 43.10 | 20.82 | 433.4724 |
| 6 | 79.87 | 52.19 | 27.68 | 766.1824 |
| 8 | 88.25 | 56.20 | 32.05 | 1027.203 |
| 10 | 91.91 | 58.17 | 33.74 | 1138.388 |
| 12 | 94.89 | 60.98 | 33.91 | 1149.888 |
| Total | 474.94 | 309.73 | 165.21 | 4695.336 |

$f_1 = 34.78$    [NMT 15]; $f_2 = 29.32$    [NLT 50]

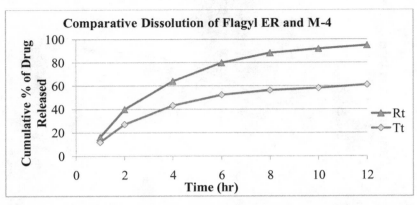

**Fig 3.49: Comparative *in vitro* Metronidazole release profile for $f_1$ and $f_2$ test: Reference is Flagyl ER tablet and test is prepared M-5**

From the above study it is seen that among formulations U-1 to U-3, U-1 and U-2 meet the specification of bioequibalance with Flagyl ER in terms of Difference Factor ($f_1$) and Similarity Factor ($f_2$). Between these U-2 was the best candidates for bioequibalance study. Again among formulations M-1 to M-5, M-2, M-3 and M-4 meet the specification of bioequibalance with Flagyl ER in terms of Difference Factor ($f_1$) and Similarity Factor ($f_2$). Between these M-3 were the best candidates for bioequibalance study.

**Table 3.22: Summary of bioequivalence analysis**

| Formulation | Difference factor ($f_1$) | Specification ($f_1$) | Similarity factor ($f_2$) | Specification ($f_2$) |
|---|---|---|---|---|
| U-1 | 10.03 | | 56.21 | |
| U-2 | 4.48 | *Not more than 15* | 70.21 | *Not less than 50* |
| U-3 | 23.93 | | 37.96 | |

| | | | | |
|---|---|---|---|---|
| M-1 | 16.38 | | 46.03 | |
| M-2 | 9.92 | | 56.49 | |
| M-3 | 4.34 | | 72.39 | |
| M-4 | 7.08 | | 61.85 | |
| M-5 | 34.78 | | 29.32 | |

Among all the proposed formulation U-2 and M-3 showed better dissolution rate from which **M-3** was suitable candidate for stability study as U-2 has poor hardness for blister packing. Moreover in bioequivalence study M-3 showed more identical release pattern in term of Difference Factor $(f_1)$ and Similarity Factor $(f_2)$ than U-2.

## 3.8 Stability Studies

For the purpose of stability study three batches were manufactured according to the proposed formulation M-3. The stability studies were carried out at $40°C \pm 2°C$ & $75$ % $RH \pm 5\%$ RH for accelerated condition in Alu – PVC blister pack according to ICH Guide line. The samples were tested initially, after three months and after six months that the stability test has been carried out up to 06 months at accelerated condition.

**Table 3.23 Accelerated Stability Study Report of Metronidazole ER Tablets at 40°C± 2°C & 75 % RH± 5% RH (1st Batch).**

| Properties | | Initial | After 3-Months | After 6-Months | Specifications |
|---|---|---|---|---|---|
| Drug Content (%) | | 98.83 | 99.12 | 99.54 | 95-105 |
| Friability (%) | | 0.21 | 0.17 | 0.23 | NMT 1 % |
| Dissolution (%) | At Start | 0.00 | 0.00 | 0.00 | 0.00 |
| | After 1 hr | 16.83 | 15.28 | 18.48 | 15-25 |
| | After 2 hrs | 40.59 | 43.22 | 46.77 | 35-50 |
| | After 4 hrs | 64.28 | 65.87 | 67.46 | 60-75 |
| | After 6 hrs | 83.11 | 84.56 | 87.70 | 75-90 |
| | After 8 hrs | 92.54 | 93.43 | 94.38 | 80-95 |
| | After 10 hrs | 94.11 | 96.12 | 98.51 | 90-100 |
| | After 12 hrs | 97.52 | 98.07 | 100.23 | NLT 90 |

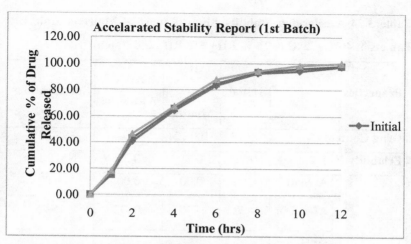

Fig 3.50 Accelerated Stability Report of 1st Batch of proposed

formulation M-3

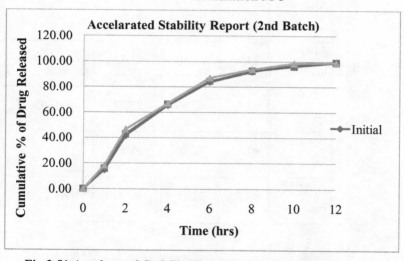

Fig 3.51 Accelerated Stability Report of 2nd Batch of proposed

formulation

**Table 3.24 Accelerated Stability Study Report of Metronidazole ER Tablets at 40°C± 2°C & 75 % RH± 5% RH (2nd Batch).**

| Properties | | Initial | After 3-Months | After 6-Months | Specifications |
|---|---|---|---|---|---|
| Drug Content (%) | | 99.13 | 100.12 | 99.14 | 95-105 |
| Friability (%) | | 0.11 | 0.21 | 0.25 | NMT 1 % |
| Dissolution (%) | At Start | 0.00 | 0.00 | 0.00 | 0.00 |
| | After 1 hr | 14.76 | 15.71 | 18.32 | 15-25 |
| | After 2 hrs | 41.38 | 42.92 | 46.54 | 35-50 |
| | After 4 hrs | 65.35 | 66.26 | 67.00 | 60-75 |
| | After 6 hrs | 83.90 | 84.50 | 87.23 | 75-90 |
| | After 8 hrs | 92.04 | 92.66 | 93.77 | 80-95 |
| | After 10 hrs | 97.76 | 96.16 | 98.54 | 90-100 |
| | After 12 hrs | 99.39 | 98.95 | 99.21 | NLT 90 |

**Table 3.25 Accelerated Stability Study Report of Metronidazole ER Tablets at 40°C± 2°C & 75 % RH± 5% RH (3rd Batch).**

| Properties | | Initial | After 3-Months | After 6-Months | Specifications |
|---|---|---|---|---|---|
| Drug Content (%) | | 98.66 | 100.12 | 100.51 | 95-105 |
| Friability (%) | | 0.19 | 0.23 | 0.21 | NMT 1 % |
| Dissolution (%) | At Start | 0.00 | 0.00 | 0.00 | 0.00 |
| | After 1 hr | 16.94 | 15.75 | 18.66 | 15-25 |
| | After 2 hrs | 43.90 | 42.61 | 45.84 | 35-50 |
| | After 4 hrs | 66.25 | 65.35 | 68.42 | 60-75 |
| | After 6 hrs | 85.03 | 84.33 | 87.67 | 75-90 |
| | After 8 hrs | 91.58 | 94.79 | 93.97 | 80-95 |
| | After 10 hrs | 98.30 | 99.13 | 99.14 | 90-100 |
| | After 12 hrs | 99.48 | 100.02 | 98.97 | NLT 90 |

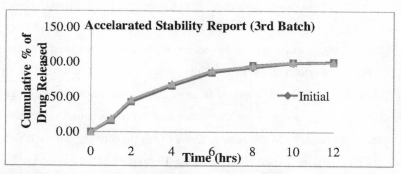

Fig 3.52 Accelerated Stability Report of 3rd Batch of proposed formulation M-3

### 3.8.1 The test results obtained at the above-mentioned condition are as follows:

- No significant change in appearance of the Tablet at accelerated condition.
- The potency of the active ingredient is in within limit at accelerated condition.
- Coating properties meet with the requirements.
- Dissolution tests are within limit at accelerated condition.
- Related substances comply with the test of BP.
- No interaction of the intermediate pack with the pharmaceutical dosage form is found during the study, proving that the Alu – PVC blister pack is suitable for the product.

### 4. Conclusion

Sustained release matrix tablets of metronidazole were prepared successfully using Eudragit NM30D and Methocel Premium K4M as polymer which retard the release and achieve required dissolution profile. The types and amounts of pharmaceutical excipients in tablets were found to crucially control metronidazole release characteristics. Release profiles of tablets change significantly with change of polymer content and polymer type. From the study it is evident that release of metronidazole from Methocel Premium K4M matrices is more controlled than from Eudragit NM30D matrices. Results were also in favor of the formulations containing Mehtocel Premium K4M matrices in terms of hardness of the tablets which was much too poor for tablets containing Eudragit NM30D matrices for blister packing. *In vitro* bioequivalence studies reveal that dissolution profile is much more identical in case of Methocel Premium K4M matrices especially in case of proposed formulation M-3 in terms of Difference Factor ($f_1$) and Similarity factor ($f_2$). Results of stability study at start, after three months and finally after six months were also very much satisfactory for all three batches in the proposed alu-alu blister packs. Integrity of all the other excepients and film coating in tablets were also satisfactory enough after six months of stability study.

So, from all concerns, from the study it is evident that proposed formulation M-3 posses all the required characteristics to provide an extended release metronidazole composition that will be stable enough and capable of delivering acceptable bioavailability for up to 24 hours.

## 5. References

- Amidon, G.L. and Löbenberg, R. 2000. Modern Bioavailability, Bioequivalence and Biopharmaceutics Classification system. New Scientific Approaches to International Regulatory Standards, *Eur. J. Pharmaceutics and Biopharmaceutic*. 50:3–12.

- Armand J.Y., Magnard. J.L. and Vernaud, J.M. 1987. Modeling of the release of drug in gastric fluid form spheric galenics from Eudragit matrix, *International J. of Pharmaceutics*. 40: 33-41

- Batycky, R.P., Hanes, J., Langer, R. and Edwardrs, D.A., 1997. A theoretical model of erosion and macromolecular drug release from biodegrading microspheres, *J Pharm Sci*. 89(12): 1464-77.

- Ballard, B.E., 1978. An overview of prolonged action drug dosage forms. In: Sustained & controlled release drug delivery systems. Edited by J.R.Robinson.NewYork, Marcel Dekker.

- BASF, 1999. Technical Information, ME 397e.

- Beren, A.R. and Hopfenberg, H.B.1978. Diffusion relaxation in glassy polymer powders: Separation of diffusion and relaxation parameters, *polymers*. 19:489.

- Bettini, R., Peppas, H., Massimo, G., Catellani, P.L., and Vitali, T., 1998. Swelling and drug release in hydrogel matrixes: Polymer viscosity and matrix porosity effects", *Eur. J. Pharm. Sci*. 2: 213-19.

- Bidah, D. and Vergnaud, J.M. 1990. Dosage forms with a polymer matrix and a swelling polymer, *Int. Journal of Ph*armac*eutics*, **77**(2-3) 81-87.

- Brazel J.G., Peck, G.H. and Peppas Y.T., 2000. Pharmaceutical granulation and tablet formulation using neural network in sustained release formulations, *J Control Release*, **26**(2): 211-215.

- British Pharmacopoeia (B.P.). 2009. Ed. Vol. 2. London, the United Kingdom: The British Pharmacopoeia Secretariat, pp.1367–1369.

- Capan. Y. 1889. Influence of technological factors on formulation of sustained release tablet, *Drug Development and Industrial pharmacy*.**15** (6): 927-956,

- Chien YW, 1992, In: Chien YW, ed: Novel drug Delivery Systems, 2nd edition, Marcel Dekker, New York, 1.

- Comets, M. F. and Sannet, H.J. 2000. Implications of pharmaceutical sciences, *Drug Dev ind Pharm.* 21 (1): 119-155,

- Dakkuri, A., Schroeder, H.G. and Deluca, P.P. 1978. Sustained release from inert matrixes II: effect of surfactants on Tripelennamine Hydrochloride release, *J. Pharm Sci.* 67: 354-357,

- Desai, S.J., Simonolli, A.P., and Higuchi,W.I., 1965. Investigation factors influencing release rate of solid drug dispersed in inert matirces, *J Pharm Sci.* 54:1459-1464.

- Dighe, S.V. and Adams, W.P. 1988. Bioavailability and bioequivalence of oral controlled release products. In: Welling PG, Tse Fis (Eds). Pharmacokinetics, Regulatory, Industrial, Academic, Perspective. pp.755-782. Marcel Dekker Inc, New York.

- Fambri, L., Migliaresi, C., Kesenci,K. and Piskin, E. 2002. Biodegradable polymers, *Integrated biomaterial sci.5:124-127*

- Fessi H., Marty, J.P., Puiseiux F. and Carstensen, J.Y. 1982. Square root of time dependence of matrix formulations with low drug content, *J. pharm Sci.*70: 714, 749-752.

- Focher B. Marzetti A., Sarto V. Balltrame P.L. and Carmitti. P 1984. Cellulosic materials: structure and enzymatic hydrolysis relationships. *J. Appl. Polym. Sci.* 29: 3329-3338

- Ford, J.L., Rubinstein, M.H. and Hogan J.E. 1989 "Study on controlled drug release kinetics from hydrophilic matrices," *Int. J. Pharm.* 40: 223 -234.

169

- Gardner C. 1983, Drug Targeting: Potentials and Limitations, In: Briemer, D.D, Speiser, P.(eds.). Topics in Pharmaceutical Science. pp. 291-303

- Giddings, A.E.B., Farquharson-Roberts, M.A. and Nunn, A.J. 1975. Perforation of small bowel due to slow release potassium chloride (slow-K), *Brit. Med.J.*,206.

- Gombotz. J, Nellore. R.V. and Pettie K., 1995. Identification of critical formulation and processing variables for metoprolol tartarate extended release tablets, *J. Control Release*. 59:327-342

- Gregoriadis, G. 1977. Targeting of Drugs Nature, 265 (3): 407-411.

- Heller, J.1984, Biodegradable polymers in controlled drug delivery CRC Crit. Rev. Therm. Drug Carrier System, 1: 39-90

- Higuchi, T. 1963. Mechanism of sustained action medication,theoretical analysis of rate of release of solid drugs dispersed in solid matrices, *J. Pharm. Sci.* 52 (12): 1145-1149.

- Hogan, J. E., 1989. Hydroxypropylmethylcellulose sustained release technology. *Drug Dev. Ind Pharm. Sci.* 15:975-999

- Hopfenberg, H.B., Paul, D.R., Harris, F.W.(eds)1976. Controlled release polymeric formulations. American chemical society, Wahsington DC, pp. 26-32

- http:// www. alza.com/alza/technologies.(Accessed on May 22, 2011)

- Juliano, K.A., Fincher, J.H. & Hastman, C.W. 1980. Timed-release tablets employing lipase-lipid-sulfamethizole systems prepared by spray congealing: *J. pharm. Sci.* 60:1709

- Kabir, A. K. L., Biswas, B. K. and Rouf, A. S. S. R. 2009. Design, Fabrication and Evaluation of Drug Release Kinetics from Aceclofenac Matrix Tablets using Hydroxypropyl Methyl Cellulose. *Dhaka Univ. J. Pharm. Sci.*, 8 (1): 23-30

- Korsmeyer, R. W., Gurny, R., Doelker, E. M., Buri, P. and Peppas, N. A. 1983. Mechanism of solute release from porous hydrophilic polymers. *Int. J. Pharm.* 15: 25-35.

- Laila, S., Haque, T., Talukder, M. M. U., Ahmed, I. Islam, M. R. and Rahman, M. H. 2009. Development of Glyceryl Monostearate Based Ciprofloxacin Hydrochloride Sustained Releae Matrix Tablet: an In Vitro Study. *Dhaka Univ. J. Pharm. Sci.,* 8 (1): 81-88.

- Langer,R. 1998. Advanced Methods of Drug Delivery Science, 254:1437-1521

- Langer, R., Cima, L.G., Tamada, J.A. and Wintermantel, E. 1990. Future directions in biomaterials. *Biomaterials,* 11(9):738-745

- Langer, R.S. and Peppas. N.A. 1981. Present and Future applications for biomaterials in controlled drug delivery systems. *Biomaterials.* 2(4):201-214

- Lee P.I. 1981. Controlled drug release from polymeric matrices involving boundaries, **In**: Lewis, D.H.(ed). Controlled Release of Pesticides and Pharmaceuticals Plenum,London. pp. 39-48

171

- Lee, P. 1980 "Diffusional release of solute from a polymeric matrix approximate analytical solutions," *J. Membr. Sci*. 7: 255-275

- Lipinsky, R. and Paronen, P. L. 1998. Reier.Dilution potential: a new perspective. *Pharm Dev Technol*. 1(2):205-212

- Liu, H., Magron, P., Bouzion, J. and Vergnaud, J.M. 1988. Spherical dosage form with a core and shell. Experiments and modeling. *Int. J. Pharm*. 45(3): 217-227

- Lonsdale, K. and Nixon, P.R. 1982. Relationship between polymer viscosity and drug release from a matrix system, *Pharm, Res*. 9(11):1501-151

- Lordi, N.G. 1987. The theory and practice of industrial pharmacy, LEA & FEBIGER Philadelphia USA, 3rd edition, pp430-456

- Madan, F.W. 1990. Rate Controlled Drug Delivery System. *Int. Pharm*. 24: 245-261.

- Michailova, V., Titeva, S., Kotsilkova, R., Krusteva, E. and Minkov, E. 2000. Water uptake and relaxation process in mixed unlimited swelling hydrogels, *Int. J. Pharm*. 209, 45-46.

- Mourya, D.K., Malviya,R., Bansal, M., and Sharma, P.K. 2010. Formulation and release characterization of Novel Monolithic hydroxyl propyl methyl cellulose matrix tablet containing metronidazole. *Int J. of Pharm. And Bio Sci*. 1(3):3-4

- Nakagami, H., Keshikawa T., Matsumura M. and Tsukamoto, H. 1991. Application of Aqueous Suspensions and Latex Dispersions of

Water-Insoluble Polymers for Tablet and Granule Coating, *Chem. Pharm. Bull.* **39** (7):1837-1842

- Nikano, M. and Rayan, P. K. 1983. Sustained Release of theophylline from hydroxypropyl methyl cellulose tablets, *J. Pharm Sci.* **72** (4): 378

- Patrick, B. O. and McGinity, J.W. 1997. Preparation of microspheres by the solvent evaporation technique, *Advanced Drug Delivery Reviews.* **28**(1):25-42

- Peppas, N.A. and Korsmeyer R.W. 1986. Hydrogels in medicine and Pharmacy, properties and application. CRC, *Boca Ralton,* **3**:109-305.

- Perkins, W.G. and Beageal, T.F. 1971. Biopharmaceutics of orally administered drugs. *Ellis Horwood, NewYork*, pp72-73

- Peterlin, A. 1979-1980. Diffusion with discontinuous swelling.VI Type II Diffusion into spherical particles, *Polym Eng,sci.* **20**:238-251,

- Potter, A. Proudfoot, S.G. Banks M. & Aulton M.E. 1992. Factors affecting dissolution controlled drug release from a compacted dry powder mix. Precidings of the 6th International Conference on Pharmaceutical Technology, Paris. pp. 90-99

- Poznansky M.J. and Juliano R.L. 1984. Biological Approaches to the Controlled Delivery of Drugs: *A Critical Review.* **36** (4): 277-236

- Qiu W. P. A. Wang, L.P. and Roberts K.L. 1988. Characterization of commercially available controlled release systems: In-vitro drug release profiles, *Drug Dev. Pharm.* **64**:123-130

173

- Quadir, M. A., Reza, M. S. and Haider, S. S. 2002. Effect of polyethylene glycols on release of diclofenac sodium from directly compressed carnauba wax matrix tablets, *J Bang Acad Sci*. **26** (1): 1-8.

- Quadir, M. A., Reza, M. S., and Haider, S. S. 2003. Comparative evaluation of plastic, hydrophobic and hydrophilic polymers as matrices for controlled-release drug delivery, *J Pharm Pharm Sci*. **6** (2): 282-291.

- Rao, R.K.V Padmalatha-Devi, K. and Buri, P. 1988 "Cellulose matrices for zero-order release of soluble drugs," In: Drug Development and Industrial Pharmacy, Vol. 14, pp. 2299-2320

- Reza, M.S., Quadir,M.A. and Haider,S.S. 2002. Development of theophylline sustained release dosage form based on Kollidon SR, *Pak J Pharm Sci*. **15**(1):63-70

- Roberts, Y. T. and Willium H.P. 1975. Evaluation of a slow release lithium carbonate formulation. *Am J Psychiatry*. **135**: 917

- Robinson, J.R., 1978 editor, Sustained And Controlled Release Drug Delivery Systems,Marcel Dekker Inc, page no –137

- Roseman, T.J. and Cardinelli, N.F., 1980.Controlled-release technologies, *J.Pharm Sci*. **59**: 353

- Rowe, C.R, Sheskey, P.J. and Owen, S.C. 2006, Handbook of pharmaceuticals excepients, 5th edn. pp385-87

- Saber, J.K. and Pulak, A.T., 1988. Controlled Release of Pendant Bioactive Materials from Acrylic Polymer Colloids., *J. Controlled Release*, **3**:87-108

- Salmon, J.L & Doelker, E. 1980. Formulation of sustained release tablets. I. Inert matrices. *Pharm, Acta helv.* **55**:174

- Saudi Food and Drug Authority, 2005. Bioequivalance requirements guidelines, Drug sector, Kingdom of Saudi Arabia. pp.2-28

- Singh P., Desai S.J., Simonelli, A.P. and Higuchi, W.I., 1988. Role of Wetting on the Rate of Drug Release from Inert Matrices., *J. Pharm. Sci.* **57**(2):217-226

- Sinha, V.R. and Khosla, L. 1998. Bioabsorbable polymers for implantable therapeutic systems. *Drug Dev Ind Pharm*, **24**(12):1129-38

- Shennan, A., Crawshaw, S. and Briley, A. 2006. "A randomised controlled trial of metronidazole for the prevention of preterm birth in women positive for cervicovaginal fetal fibronectin: the PREMET Study". *BJOG* **113** (1): 65–74

- Simms-Cendan JS. 1996. Metronidazole, *J Infect Dis.* **3**(5):153–156.

- Sutter, C.T. and Talley, P.L. and Raham, K.T. 1979. Collaborative Evaluation of a Proposed Reference Dilution Method of Susceptibility Testing of Anaerobic Bacteria, Antimicrob. *Agents Chemother.* **16**:495-502

- Tomlinson E. and Davis S.S. (Eds), 1986. Site Specific Drug Delivery, *Wiley Int., Chichester.***53**(3):13-18

- Turgut, E.H., Ozyazici, M and Rafao.J.K. 2004. Bioavailibility file:Metronidazole, *FABAD j. Pharm Sci*. **29**:29-39

- Udeala, O.K. and Aly S.A.S., 1989. Degradation Kinetics of Thiamine Hydrochloride in Directly Compressed Tablets III. Water Vapour Transmission Through Free and Applied Eudragit Films., *Drug Dev. Ind. Pharm.*, **15** (11):1797-1825

- Vandelli, M.A., Leo, E. and Fomi, F. 1995. A hydroxypropyl cellulose (HPC) system for the immediate and controlled release of diclofenac sodium. *Eur. J. Pharm. Biopharm.,* **41**(4):262

- Vazquez, M.J., Gomez-Amoza, J.L., Martinez-Pacheco, R., Souto, C. and Concheiro, A. 1995. "Relationships between drug dissolution profile and gelling agent viscosity in tablets prepared with hydroxypropyl methyl cellulose (HPMC) and sodium carboxymethyl cellulose (NaCMC) mixtures," *Drug Dev. Ind. Pharm.*, **21**:1859-74

- Welling .P.G., Monro, A.M. and Joseph, T. 1972. The pharmacokinetics of metronidazole and tinidazole in man, *Arzneim.Forsch/Drug Res*., **22**:2128-2132

- www.aerosil.com/product/aerosil (Accessed on May 23, 2011)

- www.evonik.com/product/eudragit (Accessed on May 23, 2011)

- www.colorcon.com/literature/methocel ( Accessed on May 23, 2011)

- www.mistralpharma.com (Corporate Fact Sheet, Q2 2005) ( Accessed on May 10, 2011)

## Acknowledgement

I would like to express my deep sense of gratitude to my supervisor and respected teacher, Dr. Sukalyan Kumar Kundu, Professor, Department of Pharmacy, Jahangirnagar University, for his constant supervision, keen support, enthusiastic encouragement and constructive criticism during the thesis work and write up of the thesis. His timely advice and encouragement have made it possible for me to accomplish the task as per schedule.

I am very much thankful to my honorable teacher for his animating ideas, guidance and valuable suggestions to overcome the barriers during my research work. And I am very much grateful for his untiring guidance and affection in my research work.

My heartiest gratitude to Mr. Taksim Ahmed for his suggestions and invaluable corrections in the thesis to be prepared in a book format.

This study was carried out in *SQUARE PHARMACEUTICALS LTD*, Kaliakoir, Gazipur. The members of Product Development group of Product Development Department (especially Mr. Md. Masud Rana, Executive, Product Development) deserve my strong gratitude for their friendly support and devoted help.

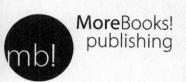
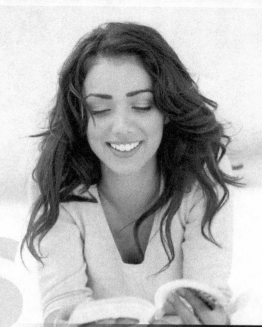